DROP A SIZE IN TWO WEEKS FLAT!

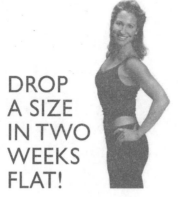

Other titles by the same author:

Body Blitz
Cut the Carbs

JOANNA HALL

with Sam Murphy

FOLLOW JOANNA'S
STARCH CURFEW® PLAN
AND LOSE FAT FAST

DROP
A SIZE
IN TWO
WEEKS
FLAT!

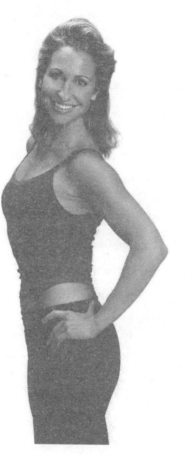

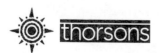

Thorsons
An Imprint of HarperCollins*Publishers*
77–85 Fulham Palace Road,
Hammersmith, London W6 8JB

The website address is: www.thorsonselement.com

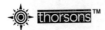

and *Thorsons* are trademarks
of HarperCollins*Publishers* Ltd

First published by Thorsons 2003

10 9 8 7 6 5 4 3 2 1

Photography by Robin Matthews

A catalogue record of this book is
available from the British Library

ISBN 0 00 713755 9

Printed and bound in Great Britain by
Martins The Printers Ltd, Berwick upon Tweed

Printed on 90gsm Talisman

CONTENTS

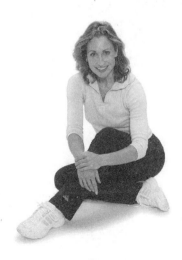

INTRODUCTION

How many times have you been on a diet? Less than five times? Ten times? More than 10? Or are you always on a diet? If dieting is a routine part of your life, you're not alone – 6 out of 10 British women are actively trying to lose weight at any one time, and there are literally hundreds of different diet plans, pills and potions out there, all promising stunning weight loss results with minimum fuss and effort. The sad truth is that 95 per cent of these weight loss efforts are unsuccessful in the long term. Yet despite all the previous failed attempts, you read about the latest quick-fix approach and think to yourself 'yes, this time it's going to work' – only to find it's just another, albeit heavily disguised, version of the 'No Air' diet.

The No Air diet! Well, think what happens when you hold your breath for as long as possible. As soon as you can't hold it any longer, you gasp in as much air as possible to make up for what you've been deprived of. It's exactly the same with dieting and getting fit – I have seen it so many times with clients. Instead of taking moderate, steady action we dive in headfirst and embrace a totally unrealistic lifestyle, only to find we go off the rails a week later. Quite simply, the No Air diet doesn't work because it is unsustainable.

Here's a typical example …

MONDAY 9 stone 10lbs – v. bad. But not for long – I'm on my fab new diet!

Felt really psyched up when I woke up. Had black coffee for breakfast, a slim soup for lunch and a low calorie pre-packed slim meal in the evening. Didn't go out after work, what's the point if I can't have a few drinks? Went to bed stomach rumbling, but feeling incredibly virtuous.

TUESDAY 9 stone 9lbs – better. Had 1 cigarette (bad – but didn't inhale).

I was exhausted today – hardly slept thanks to my rumbling tummy. Black coffee for breakfast again, a plum mid-morning and a slim soup with a rice cake for lunch – tasted like polystyrene. Succumbed to a cigarette at lunchtime just to stop myself pigging out. Feeling pretty irritable by the afternoon. Had a couple of lettuce leaves for dinner and went to bed feeling curiously close to murdering someone.

WEDNESDAY 9 stone 7lbs – good. Succumbed to 8 cigarettes, 1 bottle of wine, 2 Dairy Milk, one cod and chips – disastrous.

Oh dear! It was all going so well. I got through the morning on a couple of cigarettes with several large mugs of black coffee. Felt slightly spaced out and people at work were giving me a wide berth – I thought it was because I was a little irritable but then Kate told me my breath reeked of coffee, yuck! Treated myself to two rice cakes with my slim soup today seeing as the weight seems to be falling off but then, about 4pm, I heard the vending machine calling me. Before I knew it I'd scoffed two chocolate bars. So disillusioned was I that I stopped off at the fish and chip shop on the way home from work (well I'd blown it for today, so I thought I might as well start again tomorrow). And since the off licence was next door, I bought a bottle of Chardonnay to wash it down.

THURSDAY   9 stone 9lbs – v. bad. No cigarettes – good.

I feel so guilty – can't believe I did that. Today I made up for the damage. Again, black coffee for breakfast, a slim shake for lunch and slim soup for dinner (no rice cake). Went to bed feeling back in control but still annoyed with myself for yesterday's pig out.

FRIDAY   9 stone 9lbs – v. bad. Had 25 cigarettes, 6 gin and ton-ics and a doner kebab – v.v.bad.

Can't believe the pounds haven't dropped off after I was so good yes-terday – life's so unfair. Went out after work and meant to ask for mineral water but it came out as G and T, and since I'd got through the day on rice cakes and diet coke, the alcohol hit an empty stom-ach and had me reeling. I felt better after the second one, but then, well, I don't remember much after that.

SATURDAY   9 stone 10lbs – v. bad.

Woke up clutching a half-eaten cold kebab. Ow, my head hurts, but I'm meeting friends for lunch today – no chance of dieting there, and I'm at the cinema tonight, and can't possibly get through the film without a large popcorn and a bag of pic 'n' mix. Ah well, Monday is less than 48 hours away and that's always a good day to start …

Depressingly familiar, huh? Well the good news is that this book is about helping you break free from the weight loss spiral and achieving a slimmer, healthier body that you can maintain for life. While the 14-day plan is low in calories, it is *not* a No Air diet. It's nutritionally sound, it's varied and it won't leave you hungry. But best of all it *does* work – as our volunteers found out when they took part in our trials. Follow the 14-day *Get a Grip* plan in section one, and you'll be slipping into a smaller size in no time. But wait! It's all very well fitting into size 10 jeans or a hip-hugging wedding dress once – but if you want long-lasting effects, you need to make long-term commitments.

So here's the deal. You follow the 14-day plan in order to drop a size for your own personal deadline – but once you've achieved your goal, you promise to read on to find out how you can take the lessons you've learned and make them fit into your lifestyle. Think of the 14 days as your launch pad to a healthier lifestyle. In section two, Habit Grooving, I'll show you how to incorporate the strategies and practices you've learned into your daily life, without feeling as if diet and exercise have taken over every waking minute. It's about taking things slowly and not trying to achieve everything all at once – it takes months for an action to become a habit, so you need to take it slowly and not try to do everything at once. Eventually, healthy living will become second nature. That doesn't mean there won't be times when you just can't avoid a blow-out, resist a fattening indulgence or squeeze in an exercise session. We're all human, after all, and we have busy, unpredictable lives to lead. For this reason I've included section three, Damage Limitation, which shows you how to prevent the odd splurge from ruining all your good work.

Whatever your motivation is for losing weight fast, a forthcoming holiday, a family wedding, a party or simply the thought of fitting back into your old jeans, it doesn't matter. If it provides the impetus for you to take action then it has got to be a good thing. But sustaining that action for the rest of your life is the real key. It's not always easy, but you *can* do this, and there's no need to put your life on hold in order to achieve it. To help you towards your goals, you need information, inspiration and encouragement. You'll find all three in this book – enabling you not only to lose weight in 14 days but also to keep it off for good.

Be active!

Joanna

So you're ready to drop a size,
we need to ...

GET A
GRIP

THE 14-DAY GET A GRIP PLAN

ON YOUR MARKS

Right! We haven't got much time to spare if you're going to drop a size in 2 weeks flat, so read on to find out more about the plan and how to prepare, physically and psychologically, for the next 14 days.

WHY IS THE PLAN GOING TO WORK?

The 14-day plan combines diet and exercise. While weight loss can result from just dieting or just exercise, research has shown that a combination of both is the key to long-term results (it was also the ideal prescription for reducing blood pressure in a recent study). And it means you don't have to do either to the extreme − as both reduced energy intake and increased energy expenditure contribute to weight loss. Combining diet and exercise also helps to avoid the counterproductive changes to fat metabolism that can occur through dieting alone, according to a recent study published in the *American Journal of Clinical Nutrition*.

THE DIET PLAN

The eating plan is a carefully constructed low-calorie diet based on low glycaemic index carbohydrates, to prevent the energy highs and lows that can lead to bingeing; dietary fibre, to help you feel satisfied; essential fatty acids for a healthy heart and efficient metabolic functioning; plenty of water-packed fruit, salad and vegetables to ensure sufficient vitamin and mineral intake; and protein, essential for tissue repair, maintenance and growth.

The plan incorporates my Starch Curfew®, a strategy that restricts carbohydrate intake after 5 p.m. to help you consume nutrients at the right time of day and maximize weight loss. It also has a high content of liquid-based foods, such as soups, stews and juices, because research has shown that these leave you feeling more satiated than a drier diet, even those that involve a high water intake. In one study, women who sipped a broth before they ate lunch consumed 100 fewer calories than those who did not – and felt less hungry later in the day.

The eating plan is easy to follow and clearly explained, with options for cooking at home as well as eating on the run, and while it is a low calorie diet – providing approximately 1300 Kcals a day (1600 for men) – you can be assured that it's nutrient rich.

THE EXERCISE PLAN

Follow the 14-day eating plan and you'll soon be looking and feeling better. But for total health, vitality and successful weight loss, one crucial part of the jigsaw is still missing – exercise. Physical activity raises resting metabolism, increases calorie-hungry lean body mass and improves your body's ability to burn fat as a fuel.

For convenience and simplicity, the aerobic exercise featured in the 14-day plan is simply walking. It's not only good for your figure but your health too – recent research has shown that regular walking for as little as an hour a week is associated with lower incidence of heart disease in women. In the plan you will find that 10–30 minute bouts of walking are suggested at specific times during the day but if you really can't fit them in to your schedule, then stick to one daily walk. Some research shows that doing repeated bouts of exercise actually burns *more* calories than doing one prolonged session, due to the effect of exercise on metabolism, but the overall rule is to be as active as you can, as often as you can. There are daily step targets to aim for, to provide a guide to how much walking you need to do during the 14 days to get results. You'll need a pedometer to count the number of steps you take each day – these are available for £10–£35 from good sports shops.

The daily walking is complemented by a targeted 10-minute home routine of abdominal and core stability exercises to tone up the tummy and improve posture, all helping you to streamline your silhouette.

Alongside the walking and core exercises, try to find time to fit more 'lifestyle' activity into each of the 14 days. These are activities that can be easily incorporated into your day and don't require you to get into your gym kit and trainers. Here are some everyday tasks that will help increase calorie expenditure.

Burn 100 calories without exercising by ...

Shopping for half an hour

Gardening for 20 minutes

Dancing for 20 minutes

Making the bed 5 days a week

Walking up stairs for 10 minutes

Cooking for 40 minutes

Cleaning for 25 minutes

ARE YOU READY TO DROP A DRESS SIZE?

Before you start, get a piece of paper and write down your answers to the following questions:

- Why do you want to drop a size? Try to think of at least three reasons.
- Do you have a particular deadline or event in mind? If so, write it down.

- Why do you think you have failed with previous weight loss attempts?
- What will be different this time?
- Are you willing to add daily activity to your life? Think of three ways you could add even just a little more physical activity to your daily routine.
- How do you think being slimmer, fitter and healthier will affect your life?

Hopefully, the answers to the above questions will have helped focus your mind on the task in hand a little. Research shows that people who have an 'intrinsic' or internal motivation to achieve something are more likely to persevere than those who are motivated by 'extrinsic' rewards. For example, believing that you'll feel better about yourself if you drop a dress size is likely to help you stick with the plan more than having to lose weight for your best friend's wedding. It's important to be in the right frame of mind – positive, motivated and confident – before you start and while on the *Get a Grip* plan. That's why you'll find a positive mantra and top tip for each day of your 14-day plan. It's also equally important to be practically and physically prepared. Make sure you have 14 days in which to commit yourself fully to this programme – that means there should be no champagne-fuelled parties or candle-lit dinners in your diary. Read through the next few pages and before you start ensure you have everything you need to make the plan a success.

IS MOTHER NATURE ON YOUR SIDE?

No matter how ready and willing you are to change your body, there are natural limitations that may influence your success. I call it the 'Three M Theory' – your mother, your metabolism and your motivation.

YOUR MOTHER

The way you were brought up can have a strong influence on your relationship with food later in life. Research from Pennsylvania State University showed that women who are faddy about foods tend to subconsciously pass on their finicky ways to their daughters. If your mother actively encouraged you not to eat certain foods or not to overeat, warning that it would make you fat, you probably label foods as 'good' and 'bad' without even realizing it. If you ate a lot of sweet and sugary things as you were growing up, and your diet didn't include a variety of tastes, it is likely that you now crave calorie-dense sweet foods rather than savoury ones. Maybe your mother used to say 'finish everything on your plate' and you still do. These attitudes have taken a long time to groove into habits, and they will take a long time to diminish. This book will help you reevaluate your relationship with food, showing you how to draw up a sensible eating plan that will help you realize your weight and body fat goals, as well as providing a positive health message for your children.

YOUR METABOLISM

Research shows that from your mid-twenties onwards, metabolism begins to decline year on year. It's a sad fact that if you continue to consume the same number of calories without stepping up energy expenditure, gradual weight gain will result. In addition, there are specific times in life, for example during puberty, when fat cells are prone to get bigger and multiply. If we eat excessively during these times, it is likely that the body fat laid down in the fat cells will pose more of a problem to shift than the weight we gain at other times of our lives. This helps to explain why some friends appear to drop weight effortlessly while our own attempts require a lot more persistence. We are all designed to have fat cells, and they all have an ability to increase and decrease in size as we gain and lose weight. Appreciating this will allow you to approach this plan with a realistic picture of what you can achieve long term.

YOUR MOTIVATION

Consider this: what we weigh in seven years time will not be determined by what we do in the next seven hours, seven days or seven weeks but by what we do consistently for the next seven years. So if your initial motivation to take those first steps is to get into a little black dress in 14 days time – great! But once you've achieved that, use sections two and three to build on your success and make it last. Whatever your initial motivation to start the plan, try to find a way to translate it into a strategy that you can incorporate and build on to achieve your long-term weight and body fat goals. Establishing a strategy and action plan will be crucial, and the results that you'll see in 14 days will be the driving force to help you do so.

GET SET

This section is all about the practical stuff – what you need to buy, or have handy, how to take your current measurements (to help you gauge your results) and clear instructions on how to use the plan.

What you'll need:

- To take your current measurements you'll need a tape measure and a set of weighing scales. If you don't have weighing scales, it's relatively easy to find one in a public place – try your local leisure centre, pharmacy or doctor's surgery.
- A pedometer to monitor the number of steps you take each day during the 14-day plan (you may wish to continue using it after the 14 days, too). These are available from most sports stores or sports product mail order companies.
- A pair of good, supportive trainers or walking shoes to wear on your daily ambles.
- For the abdominal and core stability exercises, you'll need something loose and comfortable that doesn't restrict

your movement. You won't work up a sweat so don't worry about changing into workout kit unless you want to.

■ One last thing you may consider purchasing is a juicer. These can be bought fairly cheaply from most department and electrical stores and give you access to a wider (and fresher) range of juices than relying on shop-bought versions.

STORE CUPBOARD ESSENTIALS

This list serves as a general shopping list of non-perishable items that are used during the 14-day plan. There may be some other non-perishable items required for specific recipes but the list below should cover you for most eventualities.

Oils, sauces and condiments

Olive oil

Oil cooking spray

Dijon mustard

Light soy sauce

Balsamic vinegar

White wine vinegar

Curry paste

Chicken or vegetable
   stock cubes

Red pesto

Arrabbiata sauce (most
      supermarkets stock it,
      M&S is really good)

Tabasco or any hot
      pepper/chilli sauce

Tomato salsa

Mango chutney

Marmite

Peanut butter

Runny honey

Herbs and spices

Mixed herbs

Root ginger

Fresh garlic bulbs

Ground coriander

Ground cumin

Dried fruit and nuts

Sunflower seeds

Dried apricots

Unsalted almonds

Pine nuts

Cereals and cereal products

Porridge oats

Kelloggs All Bran or
Fruit 'n' Fibre

Rough oatcakes

Rice cakes

Beverages

Any herbal teas (including
Redbush) you enjoy

Soya milk

Cans

Chickpeas

Lentils

Chopped tomatoes

Anchovies

Tuna (in brine or spring
water)

Butter beans

Flageolet beans

Sweetcorn

Baked beans (reduced salt
and sugar)

Cannellini beans

Red kidney beans

Pink salmon

THE 14-DAY PLAN BASICS

Over the next few pages, you'll learn about the structure of the diet plan and how to use it. This is followed by each day of the plan clearly laid out with details of what to eat and when. You'll also find suggested 'activity zones' in which to fit your walking or home exercises. You don't *have* to exercise at these times but it certainly helps to have some idea of when you're going to, rather than just leaving it to chance.

DAILY MUST-HAVES

Each day consists of breakfast, lunch and dinner; an energy-boosting 'spruce juice'; a pre-dinner nutrient-packed 'satisfying' soup, which you should aim to eat at least half an hour before you sit down for your main meal; and a snack.

The plan also includes the following 'must-haves', which you should ensure you get each day:

- 285ml of skimmed or semi-skimmed milk (if you are having milk in one of your meals, such as on breakfast cereal, it should come from this allowance). If you dislike, or are intolerant to milk, eat a small pot of natural yoghurt daily, or take a calcium supplement.
- 2 litres of water (spread evenly throughout the day – the plan suggests an appropriate time scale)
- a multi-vitamin tablet
- five servings of fruit and vegetables (see pages 32 and 113 to find out what the best options are)

The plan has been developed to provide a balanced intake of nutrients, vitamins and minerals. The breakfast for each day is listed in the plan, while you will find the lunch options on page 71 and the selection of Starch Curfew dinners on page 80. There are lunch and dinner options for vegetarians, fish and meat eaters – try to include as much variety as possible rather than sticking with the same thing every day. If you aren't vegetarian, try to consume three portions of oily fish each week.

SPRUCE JUICES

Your mid-morning spruce juice is specifically designed to boost energy levels, stabilize blood sugar until lunch and pack a powerful nutrient punch for your body. The specific combination of vegetables and fruits has been selected to help cleanse your body and eliminate excess fluid and toxins from your body. Each juice is enough for two servings. You can either drink half in the morning and save the remaining half for your afternoon snack or you can just make half of the recipe – whatever fits in with your day. If you don't have a juicer or blender, you can opt for shop-bought juices or go to a juice bar and have one made up for you.

Celery, Beetroot and Ginger Juice

You will need a juicer for this recipe.

½ bunch celery
¼ raw beetroot
1 cherry-sized piece fresh root ginger, peeled

Juice half the celery. Add the beetroot and ginger. Follow with the remaining celery.

Tomato, Parsley and Pepper Juice

You can use a blender to make this juice.

400g can chopped tomatoes
large handful coarsely chopped parsley with stems
1 pepper, seeded and stem removed

Place the ingredients in a blender. Blend and enjoy.

Carrot, Apple and Ginger Juice

You will need a juicer for this recipe.

4 carrots
2 apples
1cm piece fresh root ginger, peeled

Combine the ingredients in a juicer.

Peach and Grape Nectar

Use a blender for this recipe.

1 large peach, pitted and coarsely chopped
2 good handfuls seedless green grapes

Blend and enjoy.

Summer Fruit Smoothie

Make this smoothie in a blender.

1 small banana, broken into chunks
1 peach, pitted and coarsely chopped
4 strawberries, washed and hulled, or use frozen strawberries
6 ice cubes
125g bottle raspberry drinking yoghurt
50g frozen low-fat vanilla yoghurt

Blitz the fruit in a blender with the ice cubes until smooth. Pour in the drinking yoghurt and blend well. Pour into long glasses and add a scoop of vanilla yoghurt to each glass.

Shop-bought alternatives:

- 150ml unsweetened ready-packed carrot juice
- 1 small can V8
- 150ml sugar- and additive-free fruit smoothie

SNACKS

When it comes to your mid-afternoon snack, we've left it up to you to choose from the list below, depending on how hungry you are and what you fancy. Each snack is approximately 100 calories.

- 1 oatcake and 1 teaspoon peanut butter
- any piece of fruit (see the list on page 32 for suggestions if you're stuck in a Granny Smith rut!)
- 20 almonds
- 8 dried apricots
- 1 small pot low-fat yoghurt and a small banana
- a palmful of sunflower and pumpkin seeds
- 2 rice cakes topped with cottage cheese
- half a small avocado filled with salsa
- 2 squares Dairy Milk chocolate (Well, we are all human!)

SATISFYING SOUPS

Both these soups are filling and tasty and they'll provide your body with some of the essential nutrients it requires. Your daily soup should be taken pre-dinner as this will fill you up and help stabilize blood sugar levels specifically when they may be starting to wane. This means you should feel more energized, less hungry and less likely to overeat at your evening meal.

Full of Goodness (FOG) Soup

Makes 1 week's worth

Choose at least five of the vegetables listed below – the more the merrier! The initial preparation and cooking takes a little while but you then have a convenient soup that will last a week in the fridge – it freezes well too.

1 onion, coarsely chopped

1 courgette, coarsely chopped

handful of green beans, cut into 1.5cm lengths

1 carrot, diced

3 sticks celery, peeled with a potato peeler to remove the ridged strands and then coarsely chopped

1 leek, coarsely chopped

¼ cauliflower, cut into small bite-size pieces

4–5 green cabbage or spring green leaves, sliced into strips

1 small bunch broccoli, washed and cut into small bite-size pieces

1 parsnip, peeled and cut into bite-size pieces
400g can cannellini beans, drained and rinsed
handful of frozen peas
handful of mange tout, diced
4–5 dried mushrooms, softened in 280ml boiling water
    (the water can be added to the soup)
4 chicken or vegetable stock cubes
good handful of fresh chopped flat leaf or curly parsley

Put all the vegetables, beans and peas into a big stock pan together with the stock cubes and 4 litres of cold water. Bring to the boil and then simmer on a very low heat, covered, for about 2 hours. Season well, halfway through cooking time.

Whizz half of the soup in a blender or liquidizer and return it to the pot. Throw in the chopped parsley and serve.

Immune-boosting Soup

Makes enough for 1 week

This is a great detoxifying soup. It will cleanse your digestive system and is packed with antioxidants to boost your immune system.

2 teaspoons olive oil
2 carrots, chopped
2 onions, chopped
4 garlic cloves, crushed
2 red peppers, seeded and chopped
1 pinch ground allspice
1 tablespoon tomato puree
3 x 400g cans chopped tomatoes
1 chicken or vegetable stock cube dissolved
   in 375ml boiling water
450ml freshly squeezed orange juice
4 tablespoons chopped fresh basil
salt and freshly ground black pepper

Heat the oil in a pan, add the carrot and onion and cook gently for 5 minutes. Add the garlic, red pepper and ground allspice and cook for a further 3–4 minutes until the vegetables are tender. Add the tomato puree, chopped tomatoes and stock and simmer for 10 minutes. Take off the heat and add the orange juice and chopped basil. Season well and serve.

A WORD ABOUT TEA, COFFEE AND ALCOHOL

Finally, try to restrict coffee and tea intake to 2 cups a day. Herbal tea or green tea may be taken in any amount. In fact, one study from the University of Geneva found that green tea could boost metabolic rate by 4 per cent. If you are a caffeine drinker, try to take your first cup of the day before you walk, and on an empty stomach, as studies have shown that caffeine enhances the utilization of fatty acids from the bloodstream, helping your body to burn fat. Alcohol is not included in the 14-day plan. Not only is it calorie-rich and nutritionally poor, it also weakens your resolve and is likely to result in cheating, snacking or going off the rails completely.

THE ABDOMINAL/CORE STABILITY EXERCISES

There are only four exercises in this home-based pro-gramme – you could always do a lot more, but these exercises are designed to help you improve your posture and streamline your abdominals in minimum time. The idea is not to give you so many exercises that it stops you getting out and achieving your daily walking targets. For best results, I'd love you to do these six days a week – a day off gives your body a chance to rest and benefit from your efforts. If at all possible, do them in the morning. Research shows that people who exercise in the morning are more likely to stick with regular activity long-term.

Do remember to warm up before you complete your exercises. In just 3–5 minutes you can mobilize your major joints and get rid of tension with brisk marching on the spot and running up and down your stairs to increase your body temperature, shoulder rolls, some side bends, full body stretches, a few squats and knee lifts to your chest.

THE RIB-HIP CONNECTION

Master this technique to see great results in your abdominal/core stability exercises. When you lie on the floor, before you begin your abdominal work, make sure you have what is known as a 'rib-hip connection'. This will help you contract the abdominals before you lift and ensure your spine is in the correct anatomical position. Here is what to do: place your thumb on your bottom ribs and your fingers on the top of the hip bone and draw these two points together with a small contraction of the abdominal muscles. Your spine should be in a neutral position. This neutral position will vary from person to person dependent upon the shape of your spine. However, there should be a small space between the floor and your back. Keep the rib-hip connection so you maintain your neutral position. You are now ready to start your abdominal work.

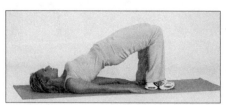

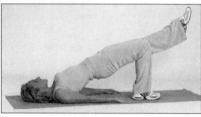

Exercise: The Bridge

What it does: Tightens your buttock muscles, flattens your abdominals and strengthens your back.

Lie on your back, knees bent, feet flat on the floor, arms at your sides. Establish your rib-hip connection and use the hips, thigh and trunk muscles to lift the pelvis off the floor until the body forms a diagonal line from your shoulders to your knees. Hold for 10 seconds. To make this exercise more challenging, extend one leg straight, hold for 4 counts and lower to the ground. Now lift the other leg, hold for 4 counts and lower to the ground. Now lower your whole body to the floor, still maintaining the rib-hip connection.

How many: Repeat 10 times

> Joanna's top tip: Visualizing pressing your knees away from your hips helps to stabilize your torso and tone your thighs.

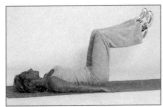

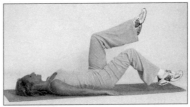

Exercise: Toe Touches

What it does: Flattens lower abdominal wall, especially the deep transverse muscle, which is crucial to target to get that flatter tummy.

Lie on your back with knees over hips and lower legs parallel to the floor. Establish your rib-hip connection. Slowly lower one leg down to the floor, dropping the heel to the floor. Keep the spine in neutral as you lift the leg back over the chest. Repeat on the other side. The trick with this exercise is to go slowly and focus on technique. To make the exercise easier, bend the leg more and lower to the floor closer to the bottom.

How many: Build up to 16 on each leg

Joanna's top tip: This is a challenging exercise. Start out trying to do a few reps with really good technique. Remember the rib-hip connection.

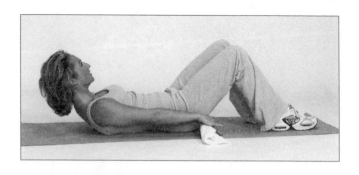

Exercise: Abdominal Curl Using a Towel

What it does: Tightens upper abdominals, especially around rib and upper waist area.

Lie on the floor, knees bent. Place a rolled towel between your bottom and your feet, slightly in front of your extended fingers. Slide the feet away from your bottom until you feel the toes start to come off the floor. Slowly curl up from the breastbone and lift your fingers over the top of the towel to touch the floor on the other side. The emphasis should be on tucking the ribs under rather than lifting up.

How many: 16–20 reps

> **Joanna's top tip:** This is especially good post-pregnancy, when the rib cage has often extended due to the growing baby. Imagine you are wearing a tight corset to help you draw down through the rib cage with each lift, but do remember to breathe.

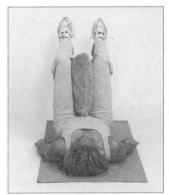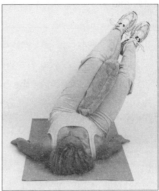

Exercise: Abdominal Pillow Rolls

What it does: Develops trunk stability and tones waist muscles.

Lie on the floor, knees bent and feet flat. Place a pillow or small cushion between your knees. Lightly squeeze the pillow between the knees as you lower your knees to one side. As you draw the knees back to a central position, focus on contracting the abdominals down to the floor and tightening the waist. To make the exercise more challenging, start with the legs lifted off the floor with the knees over the chest. Slowly lower the knees to one side but do not drop them to the floor, keep the rib-hip connection as you draw the abdominals back in and focus on tightening around your waist muscles as you come back to a flat position.

How many: 16 in total, alternating to each side

Joanna's top tip: As you draw the legs back to a central
position imagine you are wearing a belt and you need to
flatten each section of the back of the belt to the floor as
your knees move back over your body.

---

*See the Bonus Info Panels throughout the 14-day plan for trou-
bleshooting tips on walking and the abdominal exercises.*

GO!

Measure and weigh yourself at the start of day 1, in the morning *before* you eat or drink anything. Make a note of your measurements in the table below. See the guidelines on the following page for how to take the measurements precisely.

For Women	For Men
weight	weight
body fat (if known)	body fat (if known)
chest	chest
waist	waist: bellybutton contracted
navel	waist: bellybutton relaxed
hips	hips
thighs	thighs

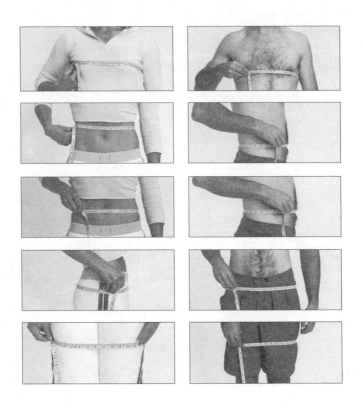

HOW TO MEASURE

Chest – measure with the tape flat across the nipple line

Waist – measure around the narrowest part of your midriff (for men, pull your tummy in for the first reading and let it go for the second)

Navel – measure around the midriff directly over the bellybutton

Hips – measure across the top of the buttock cheeks

Thighs – standing with feet together, measure 20cm up from the top of your kneecap and take a circumference measurement of your thighs.

DAY I

Today's mantra: *This is about me taking the first steps to a healthier life.*

Today's step target: 7000

Tip/testimony from volunteer: *For years I tried different slimming classes and quick-fix diets but what I really needed was education. By developing an understanding of the foods I should be avoiding and those I should be increasing, and learning to fit structured exercise around my family, I feel like I can achieve my goal at last.* **Vickie, 29**

On rising	1 glass of water plus cup of coffee, green tea or tea, or hot water and lemon
Suggested activity zone	15-minute walk (step target 1800) plus abdominal and core stability exercises (see page 22)
Breakfast	2 glasses of water breakfast cereal: 40g bran cereal or 30g bran cereal and dried fruit with 140ml semi-skimmed milk and half a cup of raspberries 1 glass apple juice
Mid-morning spruce juice	choose a juice from those listed on page 14
Suggested activity zone	15-minute walk (step target 1800)
Lunch	1 glass of water a lunch from the options suggested on pages 71–9

Mid-afternoon snack	2 glasses of water a snack from the options listed on page 17
Suggested activity zone	20-minute walk (step target 2400)
Satisfying soup	choose either the FOG or Immune-boosting Soup – make enough to last at least a few days (see page 20)
Dinner	2 glasses of water a Starch Curfew meal from the selection on pages 80–97
Suggested activity zone	10-minute walk (step target 1000)
Bedtime drink	chamomile tea, hot milk or soya milk, or hot water and lemon

TOP FRUIT

Not all fruit are created equal when it comes to cutting calories and boosting nutrients. The list below features the top water-dense fruits and what constitutes a serving of each.

Fruit	1 serving
Kiwi	2 fruits
Strawberries	large teacup
Orange	1 large
Melon (any variety)	cereal bowl
Grapefruit	large teacup
Raspberries	large teacup
Pears	1 large
Grapes	large teacup
Blueberries	large teacup

DAY 2

Today's mantra: *Every small thing I do matters.*
Today's step target: 8000
Tip/testimony from volunteer: *It was hard to fit in all the walks with my day-to-day lifestyle but I adapted the activity zones to suit my own life and made sure I fitted in as much activity as possible. I definitely feel fitter.* **Melanie, 39**

On rising	1 glass of water plus cup of coffee, green tea or tea, or hot water and lemon
Suggested activity zone	15-minute walk (step target 1800) plus abdominal and core stability exercises (see page 22)
Breakfast	2 glasses of water
	3 rye crispbread with 1 mashed banana and 25g peanut butter
	cup of tea or coffee
Mid-morning spruce juice	choose a juice from those listed on page 14
Suggested activity zone	15-minute walk (step target 1800)
Lunch	1 glass of water
	a lunch from the options suggested on pages 71–9
Mid-afternoon snack	2 glasses of water
	snack
	a snack from the options listed on page 17

Suggested activity zone	20-minute walk (step target 2500)
Satisfying soup Dinner	I bowl of FOG or Immune-boosting Soup
	2 glasses of water
	a Starch Curfew meal from the selection on pages 80–97
Suggested activity zone	15-minute walk (step target 1800–1900)
Bedtime drink	chamomile tea, hot milk or soya milk, or hot water and lemon

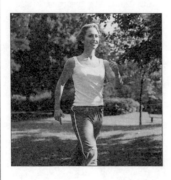

TIPS ON WALKING TECHNIQUE

Start slowly to give your body a chance to adapt to the demands of walking. Once you're in full swing, bear in mind the following tips:

- Land on your heel and roll through to push off with the forefoot
- Don't overstride – shorter, quicker strides are more natural
- Keep your abdominals gently contracted, your chest lifted and shoulders relaxed as you walk
- Swing your arms with approximately a right angle at the elbow joint, swinging them faster to speed up your walking pace.

DAY 3

Today's mantra: *I feel energized*
Today's step target: 9000
Tip/testimony from volunteer: *Read the whole day's eating plan first thing so you have time to stock up and/or make contingency plans for anything you don't like to eat or won't have time to cook.* **Sam, 33**

On rising	1 glass of water plus cup of coffee, green tea or tea, or hot water and lemon
Suggested activity zone	15-minute walk (step target 1800) plus abdominal and core stability exercises (see page 22)
Breakfast	2 glasses of water
	fruit and yoghurt: chop up 1 apple, 1 peach, 1 pear and 1 plum (or substitute 50g of red grapes for any of these), add a small pot (60g) of natural yoghurt and sprinkle with a tablespoon of sunflower seeds
Mid-morning spruce juice	choose a juice from those listed on page 14
Suggested activity zone	15-minute walk (step target 1800–2000)
Lunch	1 glass of water
	a lunch from the options suggested on pages 71–9
Mid-afternoon snack	2 glasses of water
	a snack from the options listed on page 17

Suggested activity zone	30-minute walk (step target 3600)
Satisfying soup	I bowl of FOG or Immune-boosting soup
Dinner	2 glasses of water
	a Starch Curfew meal from the selection on pages 80–97
Suggested activity zone	15-minute walk (step target 1800)
Bedtime drink	chamomile tea, hot milk or soya milk, or hot water and lemon

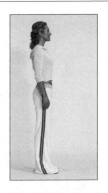

PERFECT POSTURE

The way we stand says a lot about us. It can portray our emotions as well as the general health of our bodies. Lifestyles today erode our natural ability for good posture – driving for hours or spending all day at a desk can all affect our posture. Long term, these misalignments can have a big impact on the health of our spines. Safeguarding your spine and posture does not require a large investment in terms of time.

To perfect your posture, stand with your feet hip-distance apart with your weight evenly distributed. Soften your knees as you pull up through your legs. Keep the hips square and level. Lengthen through the spine and contract the abdominals, sucking the belly button into the back of the spine as you extend tall. Drop the rib cage, pulling the lower ribs towards the pubic bone. The shoulders should be down and relaxed, so the neck is as long as possible. Breathe smoothly.

DAY 4

Today's mantra: *I feel strong and focused.*

Today's step target: 10,000

Tip/testimony from volunteer: *When you first set out to lose weight, keep as busy as possible with other things so you don't keep thinking about it – and keep out of the kitchen so you aren't tempted to open the fridge all the time!* **Robyn, 52**

On rising	1 glass of water plus cup of coffee, green tea or tea, or hot water and lemon
Suggested activity zone	15-minute walk (step target 1800–2000) plus abdominal and core stability exercises (see page 22)
Breakfast	2 glasses of water
	1 grapefruit followed by 1 slice of stoneground, wholewheat bread with a scrape of butter and marmite
Mid-morning spruce juice	choose a juice from those listed on page 14
Suggested activity zone	20-minute walk (step target 2400)
Lunch	1 glass of water
	a lunch from the options suggested on pages 71–9
Mid-afternoon snack	2 glasses of water
	a snack from the options listed on page 17

Suggested activity zone	30-minute walk (step target 3600)
Satisfying soup	1 bowl of FOG or Immune-boosting soup
Dinner	2 glasses of water
	a Starch Curfew meal from the selection on pages 80–97
Suggested activity zone	15–20-minute walk (step target 2200)
Bedtime drink	chamomile tea, hot milk or soya milk, or hot water and lemon

ABDOMINAL EXERCISE TROUBLESHOOTING

Problem: lower tummy muscles 'popping out'

Sometimes as we lift, the lower abdominal muscles can 'pop' out. This can create less stability in the lower back as well as not helping to flatten the abdominal wall. **Here are a couple of solutions to help train the abdominal wall to flatten.**

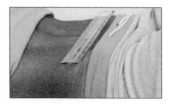 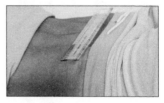

1. Check you have rib-hip connection (see page 23) then place a ruler across your lower abdominal muscles. As you lift, try to keep the ruler in place by focusing on drawing down through the lower abdominal wall – the ruler just gives you a reminder how to do this.

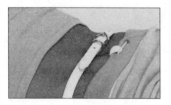 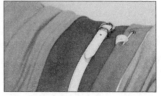

2. Wear a belt for your abdominal exercises. Buckle it so you have a little movement between your abdominals and the belt. As you lift, focus on keeping your abdominals away from the belt buckle and not pressing against it.

DAY 5

Today's mantra: *My body feels tall and poised.*
Today's step target: 10,000
Tip/testimony from volunteer: *When I first started the plan I had to completely re-think my eating habits. Towards the end of the first week I was getting to grips with it – I'd lost 3lbs and my energy levels were increasing.* **Elaine, 33**

On rising	1 glass of water plus cup of coffee, green tea or tea, or hot water and lemon
Suggested activity zone	15-minute walk (step target 1800) plus abdominal and core stability exercises (see page 22)
Breakfast	2 glasses of water
	porridge: 110g porridge oats cooked with 140ml of semi-skimmed milk and garnished with 4 chopped dried apricots
	cup of tea or coffee
Mid-morning spruce juice	choose a juice from those listed on page 14
Suggested activity zone	20-minute walk (step target 2400)
Lunch	1 glass of water
	a lunch from the options suggested on pages 71–9
Mid-afternoon snack	2 glasses of water
	a snack from the options listed on page 17

Suggested activity   30-minute walk (step target 3600)
   zone

Satisfying soup   1 bowl of FOG or Immune-boosting soup

Dinner   2 glasses of water

a Starch Curfew meal from the selection on
pages 80–97

Suggested activity   15–20-minute walk (step target 2200)
   zone

Bedtime drink   chamomile tea, hot milk or soya milk, or hot
water and lemon

STRETCHES FOR WALKING

It's important to stretch out your muscles after walking, to reduce stiffness, maintain flexibility and aid recovery. Here are some of the key stretches you may find helpful.

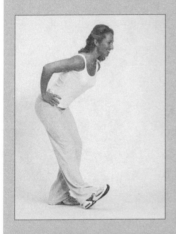

Standing Hamstring Stretch

Stand with good posture. Extend one leg out in front of you with the heel on the floor. Bend the back knee and flex forward from the hips. Make sure you contract your abdominals as you extend forward. Lift up out of the hips and check they are level. Imagine you need to balance two glasses of water on each side of your lower back to help you.

Joanna's top tip: To progress the stretch, lift your leg and rest it on a bench or low step or chair. Lift your tailbone up behind you to feel a greater stretch.

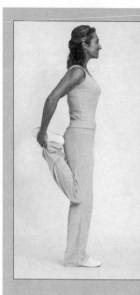

Standing Quad Stretch

Stand with good posture. Lift one leg, bending at the knee, and hold the laces of your shoe in your hand. Keep the knees together. Gently press your hips forward as you extend up through your spine.

Joanna's top tip: If you are less flexible or feel pain in your knee, rest your foot on a chair instead and press your hips forward.

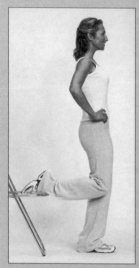

Standing Hip Flexor Stretch

Start in a lunge position. Make sure your front knee is over your ankle and your kneecap is in line with your second toe. Extend the back leg, and push the pelvis forward, use a chair for support or place both hands on the front leg.

Joanna's top tip: Keep the body upright rather than leaning forward. Drawing up through your pelvic floor muscle will help with your balance.

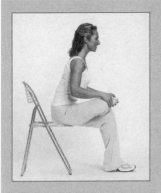

Seated Buttock Stretch

Sit on the front of a chair with good posture. Place your arms on the back of the chair, fingers pointing back. Cross one ankle and rest the leg on the other knee. To progress this stretch, place your hands on the side of the chair. Support your body weight and lift yourself off the chair, slowly lowering yourself towards the floor. You should feel a deep stretch on the buttock of the crossed leg.

Joanna's top tip: Make sure you extend through your spine as you sit. If you suffer from knee pain, try the lying buttock stretch instead.

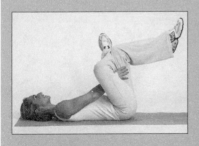

Lying Buttock and Hip Stretch

Lie on your back with neutral posture, abdominals contracted and knees bent. Cross one ankle over and rest it on your knee. You may feel a stretch in this position. To increase the stretch draw one knee into the chest, holding behind the thigh. If you are very flexible you may need to take the supporting leg slightly closer to the chest to feel the stretch.

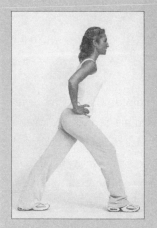

Standing Calf Stretch

Stand with good posture. Take a large step backwards, keeping both feet facing forwards and the front knee over the ankle. If you draw an imaginary line down through the middle of the kneecap it would be in line with the second toe. Press the back heel down to the floor. Make sure the body is in line from the top of your head to your back foot. Use a wall for support if you need to.

> **Joanna's top tip:** To stretch more into the lower calf, bring the back leg in a little and bend the back leg at the knee.

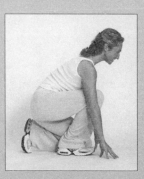

Achilles Stretch

Crouch down to place one foot on the ground and rest the other knee on the floor beside the flat foot. Keep the foot flat on the floor and lean forward over your knee until you feel a stretch on the Achilles of that foot.

> **Joanna's top tip:** Press the front knee forward and diagonally towards the floor to feel a more effective Achilles stretch. This is a good stretch to do if you are a lover of high heels!

DAY 6

Today's mantra: I _can_ do this!
Today's step target: 10,000
Tip/testimony from volunteer: _My mood was excellent while I was following the plan, which surprised me because I've always felt irritable when I've tried to lose weight before. I felt good because I was actually doing something about my weight and my health._   **Joan, 63**

On rising	1 glass of water plus cup of coffee, green tea or tea, or hot water and lemon
Suggested activity zone	15-minute walk (step target 1800) plus abdominal and core stability exercises (see page 22)
Breakfast	2 glasses of water
	baked beans on toast: warm a small can (150g) of baked beans and serve on 2 small slices of rye bread
Mid-morning spruce juice	choose a juice from those listed on page 14
Suggested activity zone	20-minute walk (step target 2400)
Lunch	1 glass of water
	a lunch from the options suggested on pages 71–9
Mid-afternoon snack	2 glasses of water
	a snack from the options listed on page 17

Suggested activity zone	30-minute walk (step target 3600)
Satisfying soup	1 bowl of FOG or Immune-boosting soup
Dinner	2 glasses of water
	a Starch Curfew meal from the selection on pages 80–97
Suggested activity zone	15–20-minute walk (step target 2200)
Bedtime drink	chamomile tea, hot milk or soya milk, or hot water and lemon

---

UNLIMITED VEGETABLES AND SALADS

All the lunches and dinners can be accompanied by as much as you want of the following vegetables or salad. Do not, however, add extra calories by stir-frying or coating them with dressing!

Choose from the following list:

asparagus	cucumber
cabbage	celery
spring greens	onions
kale	red, yellow and green
spinach	peppers
mushrooms	leeks
fennel	lettuce and all other salad
tomatoes	greens
marrow	courgettes

DAY 7

Today's mantra: *Taking action is making me feel better about myself.*

Today's step target: 7000

Tip/testimony from volunteer: *Don't be despondent if the weight doesn't come off right away. I found the real difference came during the last few days of the plan.*   **Melanie, 30**

On rising	1 glass of water plus cup of coffee, green tea or tea, or hot water and lemon
Suggested activity zone	30-minute walk (step target 3500)
Breakfast	2 glasses of water
	breakfast grill: grill 3 tomatoes and a handful of mushrooms (sprayed with oil) and serve with 1 poached egg and a slice of wholewheat toast
Mid-morning spruce juice	choose a juice from those listed on page 14
Suggested activity zone	rest
Lunch	1 glass of water
	a lunch from the options suggested on pages 71–9
Mid-afternoon snack	2 glasses of water
	a snack from the options listed on page 19

Suggested activity zone	rest
Satisfying soup	1 bowl of FOG or Immune-boosting soup
Dinner	2 glasses of water
	a Starch Curfew meal from the selection on pages 80–97
Suggested activity zone	30-minute walk (step target 3500)
Bedtime drink	chamomile tea, hot milk or soya milk, or hot water and lemon

---

THE IMPORTANCE OF REST

Did you notice that today's walking schedule is a bit easier? Everyone needs time to recover and adapt to new demands and that's why the plan incorporates this easier day. This is the perfect time to reward yourself for the hard work you've done so far with a relaxing hot bath, a massage or simply putting your feet up with a good book. You'll also feel refreshed and motivated to get back to business tomorrow.

DAY 8

Today's mantra: Today is a new day and I feel great.
Today's step target: 10,000
Tip/testimony from volunteer: *At first, my skin got worse and
I caught a cold but my spots soon vanished and I didn't have any
stomach problems, which I normally have on a regular basis. By
the end of the 14 days my stomach was much flatter and I had
lost inches.*   **Natasha, 28**

On rising	I glass of water plus cup of coffee, green tea or tea, or hot water and lemon
Suggested activity zone	15-minute walk (step target 1800) plus abdominal and core stability exercises (see page 22)
Breakfast	2 glasses of water porridge: 110g porridge oats cooked with 140ml semi-skimmed milk and garnished with 4 chopped dried apricots cup of tea or coffee
Mid-morning spruce juice	choose a juice from those listed on page 14
Suggested activity zone	20-minute walk (step target 2400)
Lunch	I glass of water a lunch from the options suggested on pages 71–9
Mid-afternoon snack	2 glasses of water a snack from the options listed on page 19

Suggested activity zone	30-minute walk (step target 3600)
Satisfying soup	1 bowl of FOG or Immune-boosting soup
Dinner	2 glasses of water
	a Starch Curfew meal from the selection on pages 80–97
Suggested activity zone	15–20-minute walk (step target 2200)
Bedtime drink	chamomile tea, hot milk or soya milk, or hot water and lemon

---

NOT BOTHERING WITH THE BEDTIME DRINK?

You may find the bedtime drink helps you sleep better and wake up refreshed. Warm fluids are more soothing than cold drinks at this time, when you want your body to relax. Milky drinks, including soya-based ones, are a good source of the amino acid tryptophan, consumption of which can boost brain serotonin levels, leaving you feeling relaxed and sleepy. Chamomile is a soothing herb, which can aid relaxation and help banish insomnia. If nothing else, your bedtime drink will add to your daily hydration.

DAY 9

Today's mantra: *I am feeling stronger and fitter.*
Today's step target: 10,000
Tip/testimony from volunteer: *Even on days when I didn't have time to fit in all the activity zones, I tried to do something – even 10 minutes is better than nothing at all.* **Sharon, 26**

On rising	1 glass of water plus cup of coffee, green tea or tea, or hot water and lemon
Suggested activity zone	15-minute walk (step target 1800) plus abdominal and core stability exercises (see page 22)
Breakfast	2 glasses of water
	fruit and yoghurt: chop up 1 apple, 1 peach, 1 pear and 1 plum (or substitute 100g of red grapes for any of these), add a small pot (60g) of natural yoghurt and sprinkle with a tablespoon of sunflower seeds
Mid-morning spruce juice	choose a juice from those listed on page 14
Suggested activity zone	20-minute walk (step target 2400)
Lunch	1 glass of water
	a lunch from the options suggested on pages 71–9
Mid-afternoon snack	2 glasses of water
	a snack from the options listed on page 19

Suggested activity zone	30-minute walk (step target 3600)
Satisfying soup	1 bowl of FOG or Immune-boosting soup
Dinner	2 glasses of water
	a Starch Curfew meal from the selection on pages 80–97
Suggested activity zone	15–20-minute walk (step target 2200)
Bedtime drink	chamomile tea, hot milk or soya milk, or hot water and lemon

ABDOMINAL WORK TROUBLESHOOTING

Problem: Neck Pain

Many people put off doing abdominal exercises as they complain of feeling neck pain. This generally relates to the fact that the abdominals are weak and the neck muscles are helping to lift the body up. **Here are two quick and simple solutions to relieve discomfort and safeguard your neck as you build up strength, tone and flatten your abdominals.**

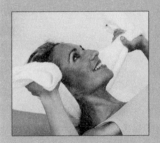

1. Take a towel and place behind the head. Hold both ends taut so it supports the neck. Keep the towel taut as you curl up and down.

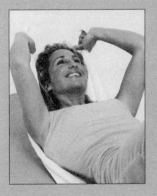

2. Place a towel open on the floor and lie on it so the back of your ribs secures the bottom of the towel to the floor. Reach your arms above your head, hold onto the ends of the towel with your hands and pull it taut as you complete your curls.

DAY 10

Today's mantra: *I feel really proud of my actions.*
Today's step target: 10,000
Tip/testimony from volunteer: *Before I started the plan, I would often feel peckish between meals and have some crisps or sweets. I've found that drinking 2 litres of water a day suppresses the need to eat when I'm not genuinely hungry. I was amazed by what this simple action did for my hunger and energy!* **Alec, 33**

On rising	1 glass of water plus cup of coffee, green tea or tea, or hot water and lemon
Suggested activity zone	15-minute walk (step target 1800) plus abdominal and core stability exercises (see page 22)
Breakfast	2 glasses of water
	1 grapefruit followed by a slice of stoneground wholewheat bread with a scrape of butter and marmite
Mid-morning spruce juice	choose a juice from those listed on page 14
Suggested activity zone	20-minute walk (step target 2400)
Lunch	1 glass of water
	a lunch from the options suggested on pages 71–9
Mid-afternoon snack	2 glasses of water
	a snack from the options listed on page 19

Suggested activity zone	30-minute walk (step target 3600)
Satisfying soup	1 bowl of FOG or Immune-boosting soup
Dinner	2 glasses of water
	a Starch Curfew meal from the selection on pages 80–97
Suggested activity zone	15–20-minute walk (step target 2200)
Bedtime drink	chamomile tea, hot milk or soya milk, or hot water and lemon

SORE SHINS?

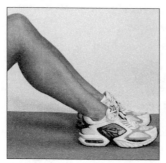 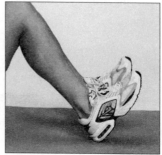

If you're not accustomed to walking, you may find that the area along the front of your shins is sore or tender, particularly if you've been walking mainly on hard surfaces like concrete. This soreness is usually a result of inflammation of the anterior tibialis muscles, which lie along the front of the shin. These muscles are often weak and are prone to inflammation when we increase their usage.

To combat this problem, try this shin strengthening exercise.

Lie on your back, knees bent, feet flat on the floor. Lift your toes off the floor, drawing them into your shins. The heels stay on the floor. Hold for 10 seconds and release. To make this harder you can attach a dynaband over the top of the foot and secure against a post as you lift your foot – you will then have the extra resistance of the band to work against.

DAY 11

Today's mantra: *I feel in control.*
Today's step target: 10,000
Tip/testimony from volunteer: *The hardest recommendation to follow for me was to exercise. I now exercise every day for at least 30 minutes, including a speed walk/jog first thing in the morning. That alone means I start the day with a strong sense of positive achievement.* **Vanessa, 55**

On rising	1 glass of water plus cup of coffee, green tea or tea, or hot water and lemon
Suggested activity zone	15-minute walk (step target 1800) plus abdominal and core stability exercises (see page 22)
Breakfast	2 glasses of water apricot and banana smoothie: soften 6 dried apricots in boiling water, then place a ripe banana, a small pot of natural yoghurt, a spoonful of honey and 140ml semi-skimmed milk into a blender, add the softened apricots and blend until smooth
Mid-morning spruce juice	choose a juice from those listed on page 14
Suggested activity zone	20-minute walk (step target 2400)
Lunch	1 glass of water a lunch from the options suggested on pages 71–9

Mid-afternoon snack	2 glasses of water
	a snack from the options listed on page 19
Suggested activity zone	30-minute walk (step target 3600)
Satisfying soup	1 bowl of FOG or Immune-boosting soup
Dinner	2 glasses of water
	a Starch Curfew meal from the selection on pages 80–97
Suggested activity zone	15–20-minute walk (step target 2200)
Bedtime drink	chamomile tea, hot milk or soya milk, or hot water and lemon

---

EAT TO GET SLIM

If you've followed the plan correctly it's likely that you haven't felt hungry. You may even have felt tempted to skip your spruce juice or miss out an afternoon snack. After all, the more calories you can cut, the better, right? Wrong! The very process of digestion actually increases your metabolism and contributes significantly – roughly 5 per cent – to your daily energy expenditure. So skipping meals and snacks denies your body the chance to rev up its metabolism in order to digest them. If you feel over-full and really don't want to eat as much as is suggested, try reducing the amounts at *all* meals rather than cutting out specific ones altogether.

DAY I2

Today's mantra: I feel like a new person!
Today's step target: I0,000
Tip/testimony from volunteer: *Don't get disheartened if, from time to time, you fail to stick with the plan. A realistic and flexible approach is just as important as being disciplined.* **Tom, 29**

On rising	I glass of water plus cup of coffee, green tea or tea, or hot water and lemon
Suggested activity zone	I5-minute walk (step target I800) plus abdominal and core stability exercises (see page 22)
Breakfast	2 glasses of water
	3 rye crispbread with I mashed banana and 25g peanut butter
	cup of tea or coffee
Mid-morning spruce juice	choose a juice from those listed on page I4
Suggested activity zone	20-minute walk (step target 2400)
Lunch	I glass of water
	a lunch from the options suggested on pages 7I–9
Mid-afternoon snack	2 glasses of water
	a snack from the options listed on page I9
Suggested activity zone	30-minute walk (step target 3600)

Satisfying soup	1 bowl of FOG or Immune-boosting soup
Dinner	2 glasses of water
	a Starch Curfew meal from the selection on pages 80–97
Suggested activity zone	15–20-minute walk (step target 2200)
Bedtime drink	chamomile tea, hot milk or soya milk, or hot water and lemon

---

EVERY STEP COUNTS

Walking is about the best exercise we can do. It is the simplest, least expensive and most effective exercise for the vast majority of individuals. The health benefits of walking have been known for a long time, but now research has quantified the number of walking steps we should be taking each day to achieve specific activity goals. It has been shown that 4000 steps a day is the minimum we should all be taking to have a positive impact on our health, whereas 7000 steps a day can positively improve our fitness levels and 10,000 steps a day can contribute to weight loss. Hopefully, you're beginning to see opportunities for quick walks throughout the day, so that you can break the 10,000 steps down into bite-size chunks.

DAY 13

Today's mantra: *I've come a long way in 2 weeks!*
Today's step target: 10,000
Tip/testimony from volunteer: *I feel so proud of what I've achieved. I feel so much more active and I'm still keeping to the diet and exercise. I have bad days, but when I do, I just get back to the plan the next day instead of giving up.*   **Tracy, 30**

On rising	1 glass of water plus cup of coffee, green tea or tea, or hot water and lemon
Suggested activity zone	15-minute walk (step target 1800)
Breakfast	2 glasses of water
	apricot and banana smoothie: soften 6 dried apricots in boiling water then place a ripe banana, a small pot of natural yoghurt, a spoonful of honey and 140ml semi-skimmed milk into a blender, add the softened apricots and blend until smooth
Mid-morning spruce juice	choose a juice from those listed on page 14
Suggested activity zone	20-minute walk (step target 2400)
Lunch	1 glass of water
	a lunch from the options suggested on pages 71–9
Mid-afternoon snack	2 glasses of water
	a snack from the options listed on page 19

Suggested activity zone	30-minute walk (step target 3600)
Satisfying soup	I bowl of FOG or Immune-boosting soup
Dinner	2 glasses of water
	a Starch Curfew meal from the selection on pages 80–97
Suggested activity zone	15–20-minute walk (step target 2200)
Bedtime drink	chamomile tea, hot milk or soya milk, or hot water and lemon

DEAR DIARY

Writing things down helps you keep track of what you're eating and also increases your awareness of your general diet and may draw your attention to shortfalls. For example, do you always feel tired mid-afternoon and succumb to a sugary snack? Do you always eat the same fruits and vegetables or do you include a wide variety of types? This information can help you shape a healthier diet. In addition, as you adopt healthier habits and reap the results, seeing it in black and white is very motivating.

DAY 14

Today's mantra: *I am keen to continue with my new healthier lifestyle.*

Today's step target: 10,000

Tip/testimony from volunteer: *Since starting this diet and exercise plan, I can't believe how much weight I've lost, how my body shape has changed and how much better I feel about myself. If everybody could have a Joanna Hall to advise and look after them I am sure the world would be a happier, slimmer and healthier place!* **Carol, 42**

On rising	1 glass of water plus cup of coffee, green tea or tea, or hot water and lemon
Suggested activity zone	15-minute walk (step target 1800) plus abdominal and core stability exercises (see page 22)
Breakfast	2 glasses of water breakfast grill: grill 3 tomatoes and a handful of mushrooms (sprayed with oil) and serve with 1 poached egg and a slice of wholewheat toast
Mid-morning spruce juice	choose a juice from those listed on page 14
Suggested activity zone	20-minute walk (step target 2400)
Lunch	1 glass of water a lunch from the options suggested on pages 71–9

Mid-afternoon snack	2 glasses of water
	a snack from the options listed on page 19
Suggested activity zone	30-minute walk (step target 3600)
Satisfying soup	1 bowl of FOG or Immune-boosting soup
Dinner	2 glasses of water
	a Starch Curfew meal from the selection on pages 80–97
Suggested activity zone	15–20-minute walk (step target 2200)
Bedtime drink	chamomile tea, hot milk or soya milk, or hot water and lemon

---

UPPING THE INTENSITY

If walking at a steady pace now feels like child's play, why not up the pace and try some intervals? Don't worry, you don't have to be an athlete to try interval training! Simply incorporate some faster bouts of power walking with your usual brisk pace. Use park benches, lampposts or even litter bins as markers to space out your intervals and make sure there's a marked difference between the pace of your fast bout and your recovery walk.

DAY 15

Congratulations on completing the 14-day plan. Chances are, you've lost weight, improved your fitness and feel healthier. Here's how our volunteers got on, along with some of the positive changes they noticed:

Sharon, 26, lost 11lbs and 4 inches
Natasha, 28, lost 2lbs and 5½ inches
Melanie, 30, lost 4lbs and 8 inches
Joan, 63, lost 6lbs and 4.5 inches
Tom, 29, lost 6½lbs and 4 inches
Tessa, 24, lost 5lbs and 4 inches
Sam, 33, lost 4lbs and 4 inches

- Clearer, brighter skin ☐
- Healthier, shinier hair ☐
- Improved digestion ☐
- More regular bowel movements ☐
- More energy ☐
- Less period pain or pre-menstrual tension ☐
- More positive outlook and greater self-confidence ☐
- Fewer headaches ☐
- Fewer colds and infections ☐
- Clearer thinking and improved mental function ☐

Why not tick the boxes next to the benefit you have enjoyed on the Get a Grip plan?

QUICK FIXES

Remember to take your measurements again today (before you have eaten or drunk anything) to see how you have fared. If necessary, check page 30 to remind yourself how to take the measurements.

Now you should be ready for your big day or event – or simply feeling ready to take on the world. To maximize the results, we've provided a few final quick fixes to make you look and feel your best.

FREE FIXES

Stand tall: Hunched over posture can add pounds to your frame. Stand tall by imagining you have a piece of thread running through your body and out of the crown of your head, which is gently pulling you upwards.

Pull it in: Being able to hold in your abdominals is a skill worth knowing. Don't suck everything in and hold your breath, though. Focus on mastering the rib-hip connection even when you are standing. Training your pelvic floor muscles will also help tone your lower abdominal muscles. To do this, take a breath into the lower rib cage and as you exhale, draw up the muscles of the pelvic floor, as if you were trying to stop yourself having a pee.

Pile it up: Wearing your hair up adds height to your overall figure and makes your face look slimmer. If you have short hair, try wearing it off your face to slim down features.

Go dark and mysterious: It's a fact – wearing black makes you look slimmer. If it drains your complexion, go for a dark colour such as chocolate brown, aubergine or charcoal grey and wear the same colour on top and bottom for a slimming effect.

CHEAP FIXES

Flush it out: Rid yourself of any excess fluid by drinking fennel or dandelion tea.

Disguise it: You can get some fantastically clever underwear these days, from tights and knickers with tummy control panels to 'bum-lifting' tights. Check out your local department store to see what's on offer.

TREAT FIXES

Get sun-kissed: A golden glow always gives a leaner look than pasty white skin. Treat yourself to a professionally applied fake tan at your local beauty salon. (If you're DIY-ing, exfoliate first to prevent smears and patches.)

Wrap it up: Indulge in an Inch Loss Wrap. While this type of treatment won't provide lasting results, it will give you a 1–2 day inch loss as a result of fluid loss. It may be just the extra confidence kick you need for your big event …

Now turn to page 101 to find out how to maintain your success for life …

GET A GRIP LUNCHES

You can choose any lunch option from the lists below. Obviously where we are at lunchtime dictates what we can eat, so the lunch options are split into shop-bought options, home options and packed lunches. All you have to do is choose ...

Note: All of the lunch options can be served with unlimited vegetables or salad from the list on page 48.

SHOP-BOUGHT LUNCH OPTIONS

- any shop-bought sandwich under 350 calories
- any shop-bought sushi under 350 calories
- any vegetable-based soup under 35 calories per 100ml, plus a small bread roll and a piece of fruit

HOME OPTIONS

Baked Potato with Tuna

One small baked potato topped with 100g can of tuna in brine or spring water mixed with some chopped red onion and cucumber and served on a bed of mixed salad leaves.

Info per serving:
Calories: 308.0
Fat: 1. 9g
Saturated Fat: 0.4g
Protein: 32.2g
Carbohydrate: 42.3g

Egg on Toast

One slice of rye toast, 2 boiled eggs with sliced grilled tomato and mushrooms brushed with olive oil and sprinkled with mixed herbs.

Info per serving:
Calories: 241.0
Fat: 12.9g
Saturated Fat: 3.0g
Protein: 11.8g
Carbohydrate: 19.5g

Tomato Soup

A bowl of fresh tomato soup (from the supermarket chiller cabinet) topped with 2 tablespoons of cottage cheese, a handful of chopped cucumber and red pepper, and quarter of a chopped ripe avocado.

Info per serving:
Calories: 242
Fat: 8.0g
Saturated Fat: 1.0g
Protein: 14.2g
Carbohydrate: 23.0g

Beans on Toast

Two small slices rye bread, toasted, topped with a small can of baked beans (150g) and ½ a small pot of cottage cheese or a tablespoon of reduced fat grated hard cheese.

Info per serving:
Calories: 296.0
Fat: 2.8g
Saturated Fat: 0.9g
Protein: 19.9g
Carbohydrate: 51.9g

The following lunch recipes serve more than 1 and can easily be broken down. Why not start the Get a Grip plan with a friend or neighbour and take it in turns to do the lunch? Support on your plan can really help your efforts.

Chicken and Sweetcorn Soup with Chilli

Serves 4

1 litre chicken stock
2 chicken breasts, skinned and cubed
1.5cm piece fresh root ginger, peeled and
   grated
½ small red chilli, seeded and finely
   chopped (optional)
1 small can sweetcorn, drained and rinsed
1 bunch spring onions, finely sliced diagonally
2 tablespoons soy sauce
salt and freshly ground black pepper
1 tablespoon fresh chopped coriander

Info per serving:
Calories: 296.0
Fat: 2.8g
Saturated Fat: 0.9g
Protein: 19.9g
Carbohydrate: 51.9g

Put the stock into a large saucepan and bring to the boil.
Add the chicken and poach until cooked through – about
5 minutes.

Add the ginger, chilli and drained sweetcorn. Stir in
the spring onions and simmer for 2 minutes. Season to
taste, sprinkle in the coriander and serve.

Joanna's top tip: You can get some great 'home-made'
style soups in the chiller cabinet of your local supermarket. There are some very tasty chicken and sweetcorn
versions – so if you are into convenience – add this to
your weekly shop.

Roasted Butter Beans with Tomatoes

Serves 4

2 teaspoons olive oil

2 × 400g cans butter beans, drained and
  rinsed

4 ripe plum tomatoes, quartered

1 tablespoon sun-dried tomato paste

1½ tablespoons balsamic vinegar

good handful of fresh coriander

salt and freshly ground black pepper

> **Info per serving:**
> Calories: 321.8
> Fat: 10.9g
> Saturated Fat: 1.3g
> Protein: 15.2g
> Carbohydrate: 42.1g

Preheat the oven to 200°C/400°F/Gas mark 6.

Heat the olive oil in a large roasting pan. Add the beans and tomatoes, stirring to coat them well with the oil. Season them with pepper only. Roast on the top shelf for 10 minutes, giving the pan a little shake halfway through.

Stir the tomato paste and vinegar into the beans and tomatoes and season to taste. Stir the coriander in gently and serve with a slice of toasted wholemeal bread or a small jacket potato.

PACKED LUNCH OPTIONS

Soup with Bread and Cheese

One small flask of Immune-boosting or Full of Goodness soup (see page 18 for recipes) with a small wholemeal roll and 25g Edam cheese.

Sandwich Options

Choose one of the following:	Add one of the following fillings or toppings:	Pile on:	Season with:
small pitta bread medium granary roll small bagel slice of wholemeal bread	tuna in brine hard-boiled egg chicken breast flavoured cottage cheese smoked salmon or canned pink salmon lean sliced ham prawns grated Edam cheese	any salad or vegetable items from the unlimited list on page 48	grainy mustard tomato salsa mango chutney marmite fromage frais reduced-fat tzatziki natural yoghurt

White Bean and Tuna Salad

Serves 6

300g fine green beans, topped and tailed
   and cut small
3 × 400g cans cannellini beans, drained and
   rinsed
I red onion, finely diced
2 tablespoons wholegrain mustard
6 tablespoons white wine vinegar
25ml olive oil
salt and freshly ground black pepper
good handful flat leaf parsley, roughly chopped
3 × 200g cans light meat tuna in brine, well drained
Bag of salad

Info per serving:
Calories: 314.0
Fat: 6.4g
Saturated Fat: 0.9g
Protein: 32.3g
Carbohydrate: 31.0g

Drop the green beans in boiling water and cook for 3–5 minutes until just cooked. Drain and rinse well in cold water. Put the cannellini beans into a bowl with the red onion. In another bowl, whisk together the mustard, vinegar and oil and season to taste. Mix into the beans and onion. Add the drained green beans and the parsley. Break the tuna up into big chunks and mix into the salad.

Joanna's top tip: This is a quick lunch to rustle up for friends – they will never know how healthy it is!

Prawn and Cucumber Salad with a Minty Dressing

Serves 2–3

½ cucumber, halved lengthways and seeded
    using a teaspoon (cucumber seeds
    make any salad very watery)
170g shelled cooked prawns
1 tablespoon chopped mint
½ teaspoon sugar
1 tablespoon boiling water
1 tablespoon white wine vinegar
1 tablespoon olive oil
salt and freshly ground black pepper
romaine lettuce leaves to serve the prawns in

> **Info per serving:**
> Calories: 202.3
> Fat: 11.8g
> Saturated Fat: 1.7g
> Protein: 18.5g
> Carbohydrate: 5.2g

Slice the cucumber halves into half moons and place in a bowl together with the prawns. Place the mint and sugar in a bowl and pour over the boiling water. Leave for 5 minutes and then stir in the vinegar and oil and season well. Add the prawns and cucumber and stir to coat well.

Arrange the lettuce on a serving plate and spoon the prawn salad on top. Serve with a slice of wholemeal bread or a jacket potato.

Red Bean and Tomato Salsa Salad

Serves 2–3

420g can red kidney beans, drained
225g tomatoes, finely chopped
½ red onion, finely chopped
rind of 1 lime, grated
juice of 2 limes
1 large ripe but firm avocado, peeled,
    stoned and diced
2 tablespoons olive oil
1 green chilli, very finely chopped
good handful of fresh coriander, finely chopped
salt and freshly ground black pepper

Info per serving:
Calories: 336.0
Fat: 19.9g
Saturated Fat: 2.8g
Protein: 10.2g
Carbohydrate: 34.9g

Put everything into a bowl and stir well. Chill until ready
to eat.

Joanna's top tip: Use rubber gloves when chopping the
green chilli or wash your hands well afterwards.

Chicken and Sun-Dried Tomato Salad

Serves 4

4 cooked, skinned chicken breasts

50g pack Black Forest ham, cut into strips

and all traces

of fat removed

50g pack pine nuts, tossed into a hot, dry

frying pan for

a few seconds until golden

200g jar sun-dried tomatoes or sun-blush tomatoes,

well drained and sliced

a handful of fresh basil leaves (optional)

bag of mixed salad leaves

> **Info per serving:**
> Calories: 300.0
> Fat: 12.0g
> Saturated Fat: 4.1g
> Protein: 33.4g
> Carbohydrate: 14.4g

For the dressing:

1 tablespoon balsamic vinegar

1 tablespoon olive oil or you can use the oil from the jar

of tomatoes

½ teaspoon Dijon mustard

salt and freshly ground black pepper

Slice the chicken breasts diagonally and arrange on a serving plate. Scatter the ham over the top, followed by the tomatoes and the pine nuts. Whisk the dressing ingredients together and drizzle over the salad. Scatter the basil over the top and serve with mixed salad leaves.

GET A GRIP STARCH CURFEW® DINNERS

All of the following meals follow my Starch Curfew® principle, which means none of them include starch – and of course they shouldn't be served with rice, potatoes, bread, pasta and so on. Instead of accompanying your meals with starch you will be filling up on vegetables, so get acquainted with the unlimited vegetables list page 48 and serve plenty with every meal. Not only will serving vegetables and salads instead of starch reduce your calorie intake, it will also make a good contribution to the minimum of five portions of fruit and vegetables you should be having each day.

You'll find more information on why my Starch Curfew® is such a successful strategy on page 108.

MEAT-BASED DISHES

Quick Honey Pork Chops

Serves 4

2 tablespoons runny honey

1 tablespoon grated fresh root ginger

1 tablespoon soy sauce

1 garlic clove, crushed

4 pork chops

Info per serving:
Calories: 302.0
Fat: 12.7g
Saturated Fat: 5.0g
Protein: 35.6g
Carbohydrate: 9.7g

Preheat grill to medium. Meanwhile, mix the honey, ginger, soy sauce and garlic together in a small bowl and set aside.

Grill the chops for 10 minutes, remove from the grill, brush the glaze over the chops and cook for another 5 minutes.

Cheater's Spicy Fillet Steaks

Serves 2

250g Ready to Cook Vegetable Selection

2 fillet steaks (approx 150g each)

300g pot fresh vegetable based pasta
   sauce such as spicy arrabbiata or
   napoletana

4 tablespoons red wine

Info per serving:
Calories: 303.0
Fat: 11.2g
Saturated Fat: 6.4g
Protein: 29.5g
Carbohydrate: 18.1g

Cook the vegetables as instructed on the packet. Heat a lightly oiled pan or griddle and sear the steaks on each side for 4 minutes.

While the steaks are cooking, put the sauce in a pan with the wine and cook through, stirring well.

Place the steaks on warm plates with the vegetables, spoon the sauce around the steaks and serve.

Quick Chicken and Chickpea Curry

Serves 4

2 onions, thinly sliced

I teaspoon light olive oil

2 tablespoons curry paste

425ml chicken stock

400g cooked chicken breast meat,
   chopped

400g can chickpeas, drained

2 x 400g cans lentils, drained

Info per serving:
Calories: 363.0
Fat: 3.0g
Saturated Fat: 2.2g
Protein: 40.9g
Carbohydrate: 42.5g

Soften the onion in the oil for 4–6 minutes. Stir in the
curry paste and cook for 2 minutes.

Add the stock, chicken and chickpeas and stir well.
Bring to the boil and cook, uncovered, for about 15 minutes until the chicken is hot and the sauce has reduced
and thickened.

Heat the lentils through in the microwave and divide
between each plate. Top with the curry and serve.

Quick Courgette Bolognese

Serves 4

1 teaspoon olive oil

1 red pepper, seeded, cored and coarsely
    chopped

450g lean minced pork

320g jar Arrabiata sauce (most supermar-
    kets stock it,

    M&S is really good)

sprinkling of freeze-dried parsley

8 courgettes, sliced lengthways with a potato peeler to
    make ribbons

Info per serving:
Calories: 385.0
Fat: 24.5g
Saturated Fat: 9.4g
Protein: 25.6g
Carbohydrate: 19.1g

Heat the oil in a pan, add the red pepper and cook for
3–4 minutes.

Add the pork and cook, stirring and breaking it up,
until it starts to brown. Drain through a sieve to remove
excess fat and return to the pan. Pour in the sauce and
add two tablespoons of water. Partly cover the pan and
cook for 15–20 minutes, stirring occasionally.

Meanwhile, cook the courgette ribbons in a pan of
boiling water for 3–4 minutes until just cooked, and
then drain. Divide between the plates and top with the
meat sauce.

Red Pesto Chicken with Cucumber Salad

Serves 4

4 skinned chicken breasts
olive oil
200ml carton half-fat crème fraiche
400g can chopped tomatoes
3 tablespoons red pesto (fresh or from a
    jar)
salt and freshly ground black pepper
fresh basil and black olives (optional)

> **Info per serving:**
> Calories: 321.3
> Fat: 18.4g
> Saturated Fat: 6.3g
> Protein: 29.6g
> Carbohydrate: 8.6g

For the cucumber salad:

½ cucumber, halved lengthways and seeded with a teaspoon
1 spring onion
Mitsukan seasoned rice wine vinegar (from any good
    supermarket)

Fry the chicken breasts in a little oil until browned.
Remove from the frying pan and place in a large saucepan
or stove-top casserole dish.

Combine the crème fraiche, tomatoes and pesto,
season and pour over the chicken.

Cover the chicken and cook over a low heat for
40 minutes.

Meanwhile, thinly slice the halved cucumber together

with the onion and put in a bowl. Pour over 2 tablespoons seasoned rice wine vinegar and mix in well. Leave for 30 minutes to allow the flavours to develop.

Serve the chicken accompanied by the cucumber salad.

FISH DISHES

Best-Ever Caesar Salad

Serves 2

2 anchovy fillets

1 large garlic clove, crushed

1 teaspoon Dijon mustard

1 teaspoon red wine vinegar

¼ teaspoon Tabasco or any hot pepper
  sauce

60ml olive oil

1 large romaine lettuce, washed, drained and torn into
  bite-size pieces

1 tablespoon freshly grated Parmesan

Info per serving:
Calories: 319.5
Fat: 29.5g
Saturated Fat: 4.3g
Protein: 7.9g
Carbohydrate: 8.4g

Mash the anchovies with the back of a fork and put into
a large bowl with the garlic, mustard, vinegar and pepper
sauce. Mix well. Slowly drizzle in the olive oil, whisking
all the time so it doesn't curdle.

Add the lettuce and cheese and toss together well.
Add salmon, smoked salmon, flaked tuna or cold boiled
eggs if desired.

Wrapped Salmon

Serves 2

Squeeze of lemon juice

4 skinless salmon fillets

100g pack prosciutto ham, all fat removed

1 pack chives

Info per serving:
Calories: 338.0
Fat: 18.4g
Saturated Fat: 4.5g
Protein: 39.3g
Carbohydrate: 2.2g

Preheat the oven to 180°C/350°F/Gas mark 5.

Squeeze a little lemon juice over the salmon fillets and wrap two slices of ham around each piece of salmon. Place in an ovenproof dish and sprinkle with snipped chives. Bake in the oven for 8–10 minutes.

Grilled Salmon with Basil and Lemon Dressing

Serves 4

4 salmon fillets
4 teaspoons extra virgin olive oil
finely grated zest and juice of ½ lemon
1 garlic clove, crushed
small handful torn basil leaves

Info per serving:
Calories: 280.3
Fat: 18.2g
Saturated Fat: 3.5g
Protein: 26.7g
Carbohydrate: 0.9g

Preheat the grill to medium. Line the grill pan with foil, lay the salmon fillets on top and grill for 5–6 minutes on each side. While they are cooking, whisk the olive oil, lemon zest and juice, garlic and basil together. Drizzle over each salmon fillet when serving.

Ratatouille and Tuna Frittata

Serves 4

2 × 400g cans ratatouille
400g can tuna in brine, well drained and
  flaked
olive oil spray
5 whole eggs
5 egg whites
50g Edam cheese, grated
salt and freshly ground black pepper

Info per serving:
Calories: 348.0
Fat: 13.0g
Saturated Fat: 6.5g
Protein: 38.7g
Carbohydrate: 14.4g

Drain most of the juice from the ratatouille.

Spray a large non-stick frying pan with olive oil and heat the pan. Add the ratatouille and flake the tuna over the top.

Beat the whole eggs and the egg whites together and season. Pour the eggs over the ratatouille and tuna. Cook over a gentle heat, lifting the edges occasionally until nearly cooked through.

Sprinkle the cheese over and finish off under a medium grill.

Tuna Teriyaki with a Lettuce and Sweet Ginger Stir-Fry

Serves 4

4 x 110g tuna steaks
1 large romaine lettuce, washed and sliced
    at 2.5cm intervals
1 tablespoon olive oil

Info per serving:
Calories: 262.0
Fat: 13.2g
Saturated Fat: 2.5g
Protein: 27.6g
Carbohydrate: 5.9g

For the marinade:
2 tablespoons Japanese soy sauce
2 tablespoons dry white wine
2 tablespoons Japanese rice vinegar or white wine vinegar

For the sauce:
1 tablespoon olive oil
2 large shallots, peeled and finely chopped
2.5cm cube fresh root ginger, peeled and grated
1 large garlic clove, crushed
1 teaspoon dark, soft brown sugar
½ teaspoon sesame oil

Preheat oven to 220°C/425°F/Gas mark 7.

Combine the marinade ingredients and pour over the tuna steaks in a shallow dish, coating them well. Cover and set aside for 30 minutes. When time is up, remove the tuna from the marinade, reserving the marinade. Place the tuna on a baking sheet lined with foil and cook in the oven for 7–10 minutes.

Fry the shallots in a tablespoon of olive oil until golden. Add the ginger and garlic and continue to cook for a further minute. Add the reserved marinade and the sugar and cook until the sugar begins to caramelize and the sauce is thick and glossy. Remove from the heat and stir in the sesame oil.

Wok-fry the lettuce over a high heat in a tablespoon of olive oil until it just begins to wilt. You may need to add a tablespoon of water or soy sauce to create some steam.

Serve the fish on top of the lettuce, with some sauce drizzled over.

VEGGIE DISHES

Crustless Vegetable and Pesto Quiche

Serves 4

1 teaspoon light olive oil

1 yellow and 1 orange pepper, seeded and
    quartered

2 courgettes, cut into chunks

2 red onions, cut into 8 wedges

4 large eggs, beaten

100ml semi-skimmed milk

2 tablespoons pesto

salt and freshly ground black pepper

Info per serving:

Calories: 184.3
Fat: 9.6g
Saturated Fat: 1.9g
Protein: 10.8g
Carbohydrate: 15.9g

Preheat the oven to 200°C/400°F/Gas mark 6.

Heat the oil in a non-stick pan, add the vegetables
and flash-fry on a high heat for 2–3minutes. Transfer the
vegetables to an ovenproof quiche dish.

In a bowl, mix together the eggs, milk, pesto and
seasoning. Pour over the vegetables and bake in the oven
for 20–30 minutes until the centre is just firm to the
touch.

Spicy Chickpea Balls with Minty Yoghurt Sauce

Serves 4

2 x 450g cans chickpeas, drained
3 garlic cloves, crushed
2 teaspoons ground coriander
2 teaspoons ground cumin
2 tablespoons fresh chopped parsley
salt and freshly ground black pepper
olive oil for frying

> **Info per serving:**
> Calories: 187.6
> Fat: 4.8g
> Ssaturated Fat: 1.6g
> Protein: 7.9g
> Carbohydrate: 29.4g

For the sauce:
300ml natural yoghurt
good handful of fresh chopped mint leaves
2 teaspoons lemon juice
salt and freshly ground black pepper

Place the chickpeas, garlic, coriander, cumin and parsley in a blender or food processor and whizz together. Season well and blend again until smooth.

Form the mixture into small patties.

Heat a little olive oil in a frying pan and fry the patties in small batches in the hot olive oil. Drain well on kitchen paper.

Combine all the ingredients for the sauce and chill.

Serve the patties with the sauce and a crisp green salad.

Flageolet Bean Casserole

Serves 4

1 teaspoon light olive oil

3 courgettes, cut into chunks

2 garlic cloves, crushed

150ml dry white wine

2 x 300g tubs fresh tomato pasta sauce

2 x 400g cans flageolet beans, drained and
    rinsed

salt and freshly ground black pepper

Info per serving:
Calories: 281.8
Fat: 5.3g
Saturated Fat: 0.8g
Protein: 13.2g
Carbohydrate: 41.1g

Heat the oil in a large frying pan and fry the courgettes
for 8 minutes over a medium–high heat, stirring often.
Add the garlic when the courgettes are almost cooked.
Add the wine and boil rapidly for 2 minutes to reduce
by half. Add the tomato sauce and beans and simmer for
5 minutes. Season to taste.

Easy Piperade

Serves 3–4

A much tastier classic French version of scrambled eggs.

1 tablespoon olive oil
2 each of red, green and yellow peppers,
    cored, seeded and sliced into strips
1 red onion, thickly sliced
2 large garlic cloves, crushed
6–8 large beaten eggs
salt and freshly ground black pepper

Info per serving:
Calories: 230.0
Fat: 12.6g
Saturated Fat: 3.3g
Protein: 13.4g
Carbohydrate: 17.5g

Heat the oil in a non-stick wok or pan and fry the peppers and onion until they begin to soften but not brown. Add the garlic and cook for a further 2 minutes.

Season the eggs well and add them to the pan, stirring them into the vegetables gently until the egg is set. Check again for seasoning and get stuck in, hot or cold!

Butter Bean, Olive and Feta Salad

Serves 4

This is a good summer salad.

4 ripe tomatoes
1 tablespoon light olive oil
juice of 1 lemon
2 x 400g cans butter beans, drained
50g black olives
1 red onion, thinly sliced
200g pack feta, cubed

Info per serving:
Calories: 337.0
Fat: 11.5g
Saturated Fat: 6.5g
Protein: 18.2g
Carbohydrate: 35.6g

Chop one of the tomatoes and blend in a food processor
or blender with the olive oil and lemon juice until fairly
smooth.

Cut the remaining tomatoes into wedges and mix
with the beans, olives, onion and feta.

Toss in the tomato dressing and serve.

Well done, you've achieved your goal,
you've dropped a size. Now it's all about …

HABIT
GROOVING

HABIT GROOVING STRATEGIES

So, it worked. Well, that's the first hurdle out the way. By now you should have lost some weight and be feeling fitter and healthier. But don't get complacent! Now, while you are feeling on top of things and the lessons of healthy eating and exercise are fresh in your mind, is the ideal time to make these strategies part of your everyday life. Remember, we had a deal – together we've proved that you *can* lose weight. You have done the Get a Grip plan. Now I want to show you how to *keep* it off. For lifelong results, there's no magic pill, just lots of small steps towards a healthier, fitter you. To help you understand these steps and help you make them part of your life, this section is divided into ten parts. Each part covers a proven strategy for successful weight control and a healthier you, with tips on how to implement it and why it works. Whether you implement all ten at once, or just address one or two a week, you'll be heading in the right direction. Come on, it's time to groove some habits …!

HABIT 1

MOVE MORE, MORE OFTEN

By now, you should have got the message that physical activity is an essential part of the weight loss equation. Exercise boosts calorie-burning muscle mass, helps raise metabolic rate and makes us feel good. Ask someone if they are physically active and most will remember how they've been tearing around all day and reply 'yes'. But think about it. OK, so you may feel 'tired' at the end of each day but is it because you were *physically* active, *mentally* active or *geographically* active? Here's an example: you wake up in the morning and think 'today I have to take the kids to school, finish off that report, get the washing done, work half a day for my job, cook the dinner and do some homework for my evening class' – and that is just the first page on your To Do list. By the end of the day you are tired because you have had a *mentally* tiring day, having to juggle and complete so many tasks. But none of these have actually involved you moving your body very much. Let's look at another scenario: this time you have to take the kids to school, drop off the dry cleaning, take a parcel to the post office, pick up a prescription from the doctor, buy your food shopping from the supermarket, pop in to see a friend who has not been well, nip into town, dash into your office, pick up the kids at 4 p.m., take Johnny to football, Elizabeth to piano, the list goes on … All of these involve being in a different place so you have been active but you have been *geographically* active – you have covered a great deal of distance but you have done it with a car, bus or public transport. You have been all over town, travelled great distances but your body has barely moved at all.

So are you geographically active, mentally active or are you actually physically active? One of the most important habits to try to groove in this book is to *move your body more often*.

Many people say they haven't got time to be active. It can certainly feel that way sometimes, but think about this … There are 24 hours in the day and let's assume we sleep and rest for 9 hours – that leaves 15 hours when we are awake and could potentially be moving our bodies. Multiply that by 7 days a week and that leaves 105 hours a week available to us to move our bodies. Even if you go to the gym three times a week for 60 minutes, that leaves 102 hours of inactivity. So, as you can see, we are expecting a great deal of change in our weight and body fat levels for our efforts, when effectively, we are only moving our bodies for a mere 3 hours a week. In fact, a study published in the journal *Nature* found that non-gym goers who were generally active in their daily lives (for example, walking instead of driving, doing manual tasks instead of paying other people to do them) were actually healthier and fitter than gym addicts who sweated it out three times a week but spent the rest of the time immersed in the convenience culture. So what about those other 165 hours? Move more, more often!

PUTTING THE MOVE MORE CONCEPT INTO PRACTICE

It's a really simple concept and it's free – it's about being creative with your available time to expend more energy without putting on your gym kit. If you can navigate your day to find opportunities to move you body, you will find it makes a big impact on your daily calorie burn and your health.

WALK THIS WAY

It's been known for a long time that walking is good for our health, but the exciting thing is that we are now able to quantify this. Studies have shown that we need to walk a minimum of 4000 steps a day to achieve minimum health, 7000 steps a day can contribute to fitness and 10,000 steps a day to weight loss. An hour's walk, five days a week, also helped women reduce their cholesterol levels significantly in a recent study. Taking 10,000 steps a day roughly equates to a calorie expenditure of 500 calories. If you manage this for seven consecutive days, that is equivalent to 3500 calories, which leaves you potentially 1lb of fat lighter. But the really good news is we can accumulate these steps right through the day. You don't have to do them all in one go. That is why in *Get a Grip* I tried to get you into the habit of taking walks throughout the day.

When I started the plan, I thought exercise was going to be a problem, as with two children, I never seem to have time to do anything for me. I take the children to school, go to work, pick the children up, take them dancing, swimming or to gymnastics, make their evening meal and then it's time for bed. When Joanna asked me to think about whether I was mentally active, geographically active or physically active, I realized that, although I'm constantly on the go, I am normally just driving from one place to another or sitting down for hours on end. I now swim whilst the children are dancing and walk while they're swimming. Now fitting in exercise isn't a problem at all.   **Carol**

TAKE A MINUTE

If you have a desk-bound job, try to get up and move your body for 60 seconds every hour. In an average working day that could be an extra 8 minutes of exercise you are currently not doing. OK, it may not sound much but if you did that five times a week that is an extra 40 minutes of physical activity that you are currently not doing. If you are able to move your body for 2 minutes each hour of the working day, that would equate to an extra 1 hour and 20 minutes of physical exercise – well worth the effort!

DON'T LABOUR SAVE, LABOUR SPEND!

We are surrounded by labour-saving devices and gadgets. You don't need to get up to switch TV channels, or answer the phone, you can stay in touch by email or mobile without getting out and about – you don't have to do washing by hand or even put any effort into mashing potatoes! An American study recently reported that using email for 5 minutes out of every hour in your working day will cause a pound of weight gain a year – that's 10lbs of surplus fat in the next decade!

All of this labour-saving is adding to our waistlines and undermining our health, so think of one labour-saving gadget you could do without and put it away – or even better, get rid of it all together. The list below provides some ideas.

ACCUMULATE ACTIVITY

You may now be a regular exerciser, but outside of your allocated training times you neglect your base physical activity levels. Accumulating physical activity through-out the day has been shown to positively improve our health and incorporating this consistently can have a big impact on the total energy we burn each day. Here are some ideas:

- Always walk up the stairs
- Leave your mobile phone in the other room, so you have to move to answer it
- Think of something you do religiously each day (such as watch a favourite TV programme or even clean your teeth!) and resolve to move your body for 5–10 minutes beforehand
- Walk for 10 minutes before buying lunch

- Walk up moving escalators
- Park the car at the farthest end of the car park
- Get off your bus a couple of stops before your usual stop and walk
- Resolve to always walk to post a letter, buy a newspaper, etc.
- Increase your walking pace by 10 per cent (see page 34)
- Walk an extra block to collect your lunch
- Walk to the next bus stop rather than the one nearest your home
- Don't email colleagues in the building – get up and talk to them
- When you are shopping, only use a trolley if it's absolutely necessary. Otherwise carry it in a basket
- Do 10 squats or counter push-ups every time you are waiting for the kettle to boil
- Stand up on the train or tube rather than sitting

The great thing about physical activity is that it can be achieved without you having to put on your gym kit. While there are certainly good reasons to do structured exercise (see point 3), if you get into the habit of being more physically active on a daily basis you will find it a great support strategy when life becomes a little too hectic to stick with your structured exercise sessions. Remember, our ancestors didn't have gyms and they were far fitter and slimmer than we are!

HABIT 2

OPERATE THE STARCH CURFEW

When you started the *Get a Grip* plan, you may have found the Starch Curfew, which effectively limits carbohydrate intake, a surprising strategy. After all, we've been told for years that carbohydrate is the nutrient of choice when it comes to health and weight control. But think about it: if the low-fat, high carbohydrate diet was the solution, obesity levels would surely have fallen, not risen, over the last couple of decades. The problem is, we've come to believe that as long as we don't *eat* fat, we won't *get* fat — and that simply isn't the case. Too much of the wrong type of carbohydrate plays havoc with metabolism and blood sugar levels, which has a knock-on effect on satiety. Dr Walter Willett, chair of the department of nutrition at the Harvard School of Public Health, points out that we shouldn't be thinking of cutting out carbohydrates but simply being more choosy about the type of carbohydrate we eat. Initially, this can feel like a difficult strategy to take on. After all, most of us are accustomed to eating pasta, potatoes or rice with our evening meal. But if you're anything like our volunteers, you probably found that not only did you get used to starch-free dinners but you also lost weight, gained energy and didn't feel hungry. To understand how Starch Curfew works, you need to know a little about what happens when you eat carbohydrates. When we eat, carbohydrates are broken down to small useable units of glucose. First, glucose is released into the bloodstream, signalling the pancreas to produce the hormone insulin. Insulin takes some of the glucose to cells to give them immediate energy. It changes the rest of the glucose into a substance called glycogen, which is transported to the liver and muscles for short-term storage and then converted to fat if it is not needed.

This process works well when blood sugar is released slowly into the bloodstream, but if you eat the kind of carbohydrates that quickly convert to glucose, a high concentration of insulin is released. This causes blood sugar to drop suddenly, causing fatigue and cravings for more carbohydrates. The speed with which a carbohydrate causes a rise in blood sugar is measured by the Glycaemic Index. The Glycaemic Index ranks foods between 1 and 100 dependent upon their effect on raising blood sugar levels. The higher a food's GI rating, the faster blood sugar levels are raised and released into the bloodstream. Low GI foods, such as pulses, release sugar slowly into the bloodstream, keeping you satisfied for longer and preventing energy highs and lows. All of which helps you to stop craving sweet sugary snacks and keep hunger pangs at bay. The slower digestion and the more gradual rise and fall in blood sugar levels resulting from eating low glycaemic index foods make them a healthier choice. A study from Harvard University's School of Public Health found that low GI diets are associated with a lower

Low GI 50 or under	Moderate GI 50–70	High GI 70 and over
Yoghurt	Brown rice	White rice
Lentils	Banana	Pasta (all types)
Apples	Sweetcorn	Cornflakes
Kelloggs All-Bran	Cous Cous	White bread
		Shredded wheat
Porridge	Honey	and Weetabix
Butter beans,	Sweet potato	Bagel
kidney beans		Parsnips, carrots,
Chick peas	Stoneground	baked potato
	wholewheat bread	Sports drinks
Milk	Oatcakes	French Fries
Dried apricots	Raisins	Watermelon

risk of Type II diabetes and heart disease, while Australian scientists are so convinced of the importance of the glycaemic index that they have persuaded the government to include it on food labels. A healthy diet doesn't mean only eating low GI foods, as many other factors (such as the amount of the food you eat, the amount of protein and fat you eat with it and the presence of fibre) also influence your overall blood sugar response. But try to include more low GI foods in your diet and fewer high GI foods and you'll soon see and feel a big difference in your energy levels. And by operating Starch Curfew, you'll see and feel a big difference in how your clothes fit. Use the chart opposite to help you get the right balance.

Most people know that the disease diabetes involves too much sugar in the blood and either not enough insulin to deal with it, or a failure in the insulin's ability to remove it. But did you know that, as we get older, insulin sensitivity decreases even in non-diabetics? There is some evidence that suggests that if you eat a lot of high glycaemic index carbohydrate foods, you become insensitive (or 'resistant') to insulin and your body has to keep pumping out insulin, which, instead of converting the glucose into energy, turns it into fat. The various effects of this insulin resistance – 'below-the-belt' fat accumulation, high concentration of blood fats, high blood pressure and an increased risk of heart disease – have been termed Syndrome X. Developing the starch curfew habit helps you control your insulin levels, which in turn helps you stabilize your energy levels and reduce the risk of potential health problems.

You may be wondering if, with all the pitfalls of eating the wrong types of carbohydrate, it might be better just to stick with protein. The answer is no! High protein and very low carbohydrate diets aim to put the body in a state of ketosis. Ketosis means the body burns protein instead of carbohydrate for fuel. This approach is not supported by mainstream medical and nutritional establishment – in fact, the American Heart Association has actually put out a position statement condemning a high intake of protein as it increases blood cholesterol associated with heart disease and kidney disease. Starch Curfew allows you to apply a moderate approach to your eating, getting the balance right to fuel your energy and help you lose weight.

Following Starch Curfew has three benefits:

1. It cuts down calories without the calorie counting
By cutting out bread, pasta, rice, potatoes and cereal after 5 p.m. you will naturally be cutting down your calories. But since you'll be filling up on more fruit and vegetables, lean meat, fish and slow-releasing energy-providing pulses, you won't feel hungry.

2. It boosts your energy
The starch curfew helps you get a better balance of nutrients. You will be eating more slow-releasing carbohydrates, which directly impact your energy levels and keep them steady. As you will be eating more fruit and vegetables, you will boost your intake of essential vitamins and minerals. You may think you already eat enough fruit and vegetables, but have a read of Richard's situation:

Before I discovered Starch Curfew I was convinced I was eating enough fruit and veg – I'd have muesli and toast for breakfast, a tuna and lettuce sandwich at lunch and an apple when I was feeling holy in the afternoon – though more often than not it was an apple Danish (well that was a fruit, wasn't it) and then pasta or risotto with a bit of salad or broccoli when I got home. My wife is an excellent cook, so I thought the fruit in my muesli and the lettuce leaf in my sarnie, and maybe the token few peas in my risotto was enough! I actually discovered I was only hitting an average of two of my five suggested servings of fruit and veg a day. I knew about the link between fruit and veg intake and cancer – but I was sure I was fine! Once I started the Starch Curfew not only did I lose weight and feel fuller but I actually increased the amount of fruit and veg I ate without having to try too hard. It's so simple; it really worked for me. My wife does not have to cook me a different meal – it fits in with the rest of my family and I find it really effective as a businessman having so many lunches and dinners out.   **Richard 46, who lost 5 inches off his waist and dropped 10lbs**

To see what makes a portion of fruit or veg, check out the list below.

Salad, vegetables and fruit – what makes one serving?
- 10 asparagus spears
- 3 spears of broccoli or cauliflower
- 8 Brussels sprouts
- 3 sticks of celery
- half a courgette
- 1 large tomato
- half a cucumber
- 1 small avocado

- medium bowl of lettuce
- I apple, orange, banana, pear, peach
- I large slice of melon, pineapple
- 4 dried apricots
- I cup berries

3. It reduces bloating

Excess starch intake can leave you feeling heavy and bloated. It's not surprising, when you understand that for every unit of glycogen (the storage form that carbohydrate takes in the body), you need to have 3 units of water with which to store it. Think of it this way – if you eat a cereal bowl serving of pasta your body has to hold onto three bowls of water to be able to convert the starch to glycogen to be stored. That's not to say we don't need glycogen – it is an essential fuel – but since we can only store a limited amount, if we are not burning it through regular exercise, it will be converted and stored as fat.

Refraining from eating carbohydrates after 5 o'clock has made an enormous difference to my life. I can hardly believe it. I no longer wake up in the middle of the night with a feeling of bloat and discomfort in my stomach, my digestion has improved and I feel so much better in myself. Starch curfew is not a diet, it's a lifestyle – I have never found an eating plan that so well suits my age group. I no longer suffer mood swings, I have loads more energy and I have really lost inches. My husband cannot believe it. I felt so much better that I told all my friends and they have felt the same, too. **Vanessa, 55 (lost 6 inches)**

PUTTING STARCH CURFEW INTO PRACTICE

Here are some tips to help you.

VEG UP

Think fresh, frozen and canned vegetables. Religiously walk down the fruit and vegetable aisles and fill that trolley – whether it's fresh, frozen or canned fruit and veg, they all have their place!

At first, I was afraid my shopping budget would increase with buying all that fruit and veg. I'm a single mum, so for me every penny counts, even though I was really keen to get back in shape after the birth of my daughter. I found by following the starch curfew I had more energy – I stopped buying so many biscuits and fillers to have in the afternoon to keep my energy levels up and my shopping bill actually went down, week in, week out – which was great! I even had some pennies to buy myself some clothes to celebrate all the inches I lost! **Emmaline, 28**

KEEP YOUR FINGER ON THE PULSE

If your idea of salad is a few lettuce leaves and a slice of tomato, think again. Salads can be spiced up with all kinds of things, from pine nuts and pumpkin seeds to finely chopped chillies, grilled mushrooms, sun-dried tomatoes, red kidney beans ... Be adventurous!

I'm so much more imaginative now with my salads – they become a meal in their own right, that way I do not feel deprived. I really like to steam vegetables and add them to mixed salad leaves. One of my favourites is to steam broccoli, asparagus and mange tout, run them under a cold tap to stop them overcooking, and throw in a big bag of salad leaves. I then dry-fry a large punnet of button mushrooms in a little Thai sweet chilli sauce and stir through the cooked and raw salad – it's really tasty, so simple and quick.
Carol, 44 (lost 10lbs)

TRICK YOURSELF

If you feel a plate of dinner just doesn't look right without a heap of rice pasta or potatoes, kid yourself by getting creative with presentation. Try cutting stir-fried courgettes into ribbons and laying your meat or fish on top of that or puree or mash veg as if they were potato. For more ideas see the recipe for Quick Courgette Bolognaise on page 84.

HABIT 3

TAKE STRUCTURED EXERCISE

As you have now learned, exercise doesn't have to involve a pair of trainers and an expensive gym membership. In *Move More, More Often* (page 102) there are plenty of ideas about fitting more daily activity into your life. But for optimum weight loss results, your best body shape and improved fitness, the ideal is to combine daily physical activity with regular structured exercise sessions. Health authorities recommend that to maintain health, we exercise at a low to moderate intensity for half an hour on most days of the week. For fitness gains, the intensity needs to be higher, which is why the American College of Sports Medicine recommends exercising more vigorously for 20–50 minutes, at least twice a week, alongside the more moderate activity. You should be working at a level that is intense enough to make you feel breathless and hot. Anything from step aerobics to salsa dancing counts! Here's how thrice-weekly sessions of your favourite activity can add up to some serious calorie expenditure ...

Structured exercise to burn 1000 calories

3 x 45 minutes in-line skating

3 x 40 minutes jogging (12-minute miles)

3 x 40 minutes cycling

3 x 1 hour 20 minutes brisk walking

3 x 1 hour low impact aerobics

3 x 40 minutes tennis

PUTTING STRUCTURED EXERCISE INTO PRACTICE

- Pick an activity that you enjoy, not the one you think will burn the most calories.

- Sign up for a beginner's course in a dance class or sports activity – that way, you'll feel less intimidated and you'll be at the same level as everyone else.

- Write your workout dates and times in your diary as if they were an appointment, so that you don't end up crowding them out of your schedule.

- Be prepared – if your kit is clean and packed, you'll be much more likely to go for a workout than if you have to hunt through the laundry basket for something to wear.

- Go with a friend. Not only does it provide moral support it also reduces the risk of you bailing out, as you'll be letting your friend down, too.

MUSCLING IN

Aerobic exercise – such as walking, jogging or swimming – is the most important type of activity for your health but resistance, or strength, training also plays a key role in weight control and in determining your body shape. Basal metabolic rate – the rate at which we burn calories at rest – begins to decline from 25–30 years of age, along with the volume of lean muscle tissue that we have. The result is an overall loss in metabolically-active tissue and a gain in highly inactive adipose – or fatty – tissue. One pound of muscle requires approximately 35 calories per day simply to function, while a pound of fat needs just *one or two* calories. So you can see that by increasing lean body mass through resistance training, this depressing shift in body composition can be reversed. An American study found that 12 weeks of regular resistance training resulted in a loss of 4lbs of body fat and a gain of 3lbs of lean muscle tissue. With regular practice, not only will you become a more efficient calorie-burning machine, you'll also look more toned, shapely and firm. You don't have to join a gym to do resistance training – you can use your own body weight as resistance, or use dumbbells or household items, such as cans or water bottles, at home. Why not get started by following the Total Body Solution workout overleaf?

THE TOTAL BODY SOLUTION

This 15-minute workout blitzes the whole body – helping you to streamline muscles, tone up and boost your metabolic rate by increasing your lean muscle mass. Each of the six exercises will provide two great benefits in one simple move. Ideally, I'd love you to complete the Total Body workout on non-consecutive days e.g. Tuesday, Thursday, Saturday, Monday – that way your body gets a chance to rest, you are not exercising all the time and you get better results in the long-term. The workouts below cater for different levels so you can progress as your fitness and body tone increases. Remember to start out slowly, as studies have shown if you are too gung ho, motivation can quickly wane. If you think you can commit to doing the workout three times a week – that is great, but you need to be 90 per cent confident you will be able to complete it three times. If not – let's aim for twice and appreciate the fact that you have made time in your busy day to do it – congratulate yourself for that and feel good about it, not bad that you have not been able to do three.

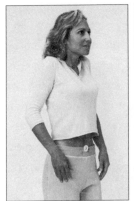
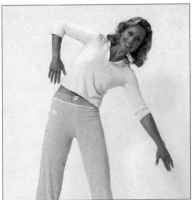
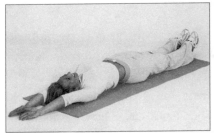
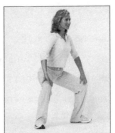
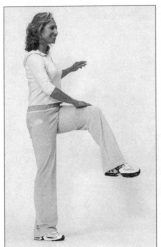
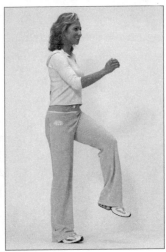

THE EXERCISES

There are two levels, beginners and intermediates. Choose which one suits you and your level of fitness and experience. Complete one circuit by doing each exercise for the number of repetitions or amount of time stated in the exercise. Then perform the circuit again. Focus on slow, controlled movements to get the best body benefits. Remember to complete a warm up and cool down before and after your workout.

WARMING UP

Before any exercise session it is important to warm up, to get your mind and body ready for your Total Body Solution workout. Don't skip it, thinking this will save you time – this is false economy. Even with as little as 3–5 minutes you can mobilize your major joints and relieve tension from your day – try shoulder rolls, some side bends and full body stretches, a few squats, knee lifts to your chest, brisk marching on the spot and running up and down your stairs to increase your body temperature.

LEVEL ONE

Start with this workout if you are new to exercise or have had a break – you can always move on to level two if you feel it was too easy for you. Focus on good form and avoid rushing the exercises.

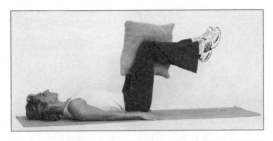

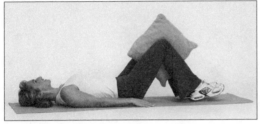

Body bit: Torso

The exercise: Double leg drops

What it does: Flattens the abdominals

Extra Body bit solution: Tones inner thighs

Lie on your back with a cushion between your legs, knees over chest. Keep the abdominals contracted and spine in a neutral position as you drop the legs to the floor so the toes lightly touch it. Continue for 60 seconds.

> _Joanna's top tip_: Remember to check out the rib-hip connection on page 23 of _Get a Grip_ to help you with your technique.

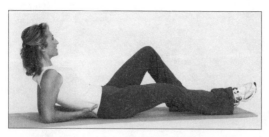

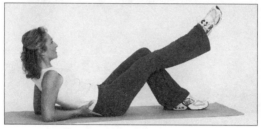

Body bit: Legs

The exercise: Inner thigh lift with leg press

What it does: Tones inner thighs

Extra Body bit solution: Streamlines whole thigh and helps strengthen weak knees

Lie on your back supported on your elbows, one leg straight and rotated out at the hip, the other leg bent. Soften the straight leg at the knee and lift it level to the height of the other knee then lower. Lead from the inner thigh. Repeat 8 times and then hold the leg up and bring the ankle of the working leg into the knee and press away again. Repeat 8 times.

> *Joanna's top tip:* Keep the foot of the extended leg relaxed, this is important as it helps target the inner thigh muscles more.

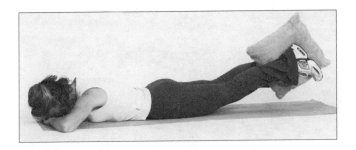

Body bit: Bottom

The exercise: Prone cushion lift
What it does: Tightens buttocks
Extra Body bit solution: Stabilizes your spine and tones your abdominals

Lie face down and place a small cushion between your ankles. Rest your forehead on your hands and pull in your abdominals to support your spine. Extend the legs and press the whole of the inner legs together as you squeeze the cushion between the ankles. Slowly and smoothly, lift your feet and legs about 6 inches off the floor and then slowly lower them to the ground. Continue for 60 seconds.

> *Joanna's top tip:* Make sure you extend the legs as long as possible as you lift them up off the floor. This helps to stabilize and build a strong spine and contract your buttock muscles more effectively.

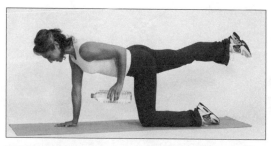

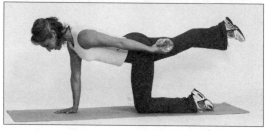

Body bit: Chest and arms

The exercise: Kneeling triceps kickback

What it does: Streamlines backs of arms and tones trunk muscles

Extra Body bit solution: Streamlines torso

On all fours, extend your left leg straight behind you. Keep abdominals contracted as you maintain a neutral spine. Hold a 2–3kg weight in your right hand (or a 1–1.5 litre bottle of water) and hold elbow close to your side, palm facing the mid-line of body. Keep the elbow fixed as you extend the elbow back in line with the body. Rotate the palm towards the ceiling as your straighten the arm. Continue for 60 seconds, alternating arms and legs.

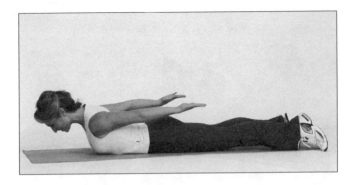

Body bit: Back

The exercise: Back extension with arm lift
What it does: Tones and strengthens back
Extra Body bit solution: Streamlines back of arms

Lie face down, fingers resting by your side. Keep the abdominals contracted as you slowly lift the upper body off the floor. Keep the eye line down. Slowly lift the arms straight up, reaching your fingers to your feet. Lower the arms down and then lower the upper body down to the floor. Continue for 60 seconds.

> Joanna's top tip: If you find this exercise too challenging, build up to it by keeping the hands on the floor.

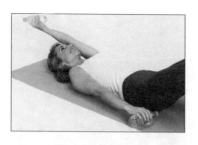

Body bit: Arms

The exercise: Scissor arms
What it does: Streamlines the troublesome back of arm area and helps you reclaim your waist!

Extra Body bit solution: Helps draw the ribs together — particularly important post-pregnancy

Lie on your back, arms extended directly over eye line. Hold one small weight — such as a can of tomatoes, a 2kg hand weight, or water bottle — in each hand. Slowly take four counts to lower arms in opposite directions, one back over the head and the other towards the thighs. Keep the weight off the floor, lengthen through the arm as you lower and keep the wrists in a neutral position. Draw the arms back over your eye line and scissor in other direction. Do 8 full range movements and then hold one arm level with the ears and lift about 5cm slowly up and down 8 times. Repeat on the other side.

Joanna's top tip: This is a very subtle exercise but if you get the technique right it really tones the back of the arm. Avoid gripping the weight too tightly as this takes the emphasis away from the targeted muscle.

LEVEL TWO

This is a more challenging level – when you start out, why not try to complete just one set of 60 seconds of each exercise for three weeks and then progress on to two sets of 60 seconds.

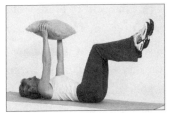

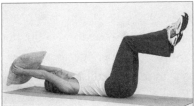

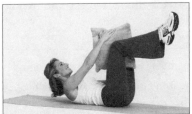

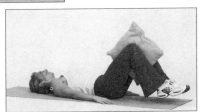

Body bit: Abdominals

The exercise: Ab combo

What it does: Flattens abdominals, lengthens torso and increases mobility of spine and shoulders

Extra Body bit solution: Targets the legs as well as flattening whole of abdominal area and streamlining midriff

Lie on your back, knees bent, feet flat on the floor. Hold a cushion in your hands directly over your head. Slowly lower your arms over your head. Keep the ribs drawn in. Lift the arms back over the head and curl up from the breastbone to perform an abdominal curl as you lift your legs off the floor. Now place the cushion between your knees. Lower your torso back down to the floor and slowly lower your toes to the floor. Imagine the floor is covered in superglue to avoid you resting your feet on the floor. Draw the legs back into the chest, curling up through the upper body to take hold of the cushion once again. Lower the legs to the floor. Repeat the whole sequence.

> Joanna's top tip: Remember to keep the abdominals contracted and the spine in neutral position as you drop the legs to the floor, so the toes lightly touch.

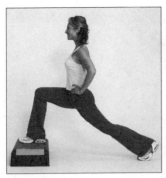 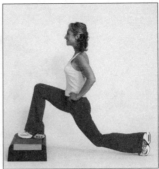

Body bit: Legs

The exercise: Four point lunge

What it does: Shapes and strengthens thighs and gluteals

Extra Body bit solution: The large number of muscles used in this exercise burns extra calories

Stand on a low bench or bottom stair. Extend one leg back with a large stride so the leg has only a slight bend at the knee, lower the knee of the extended leg towards the floor, straighten the leg and bring the extended leg back to the start position. Change sides.

> *Joanna's top tip:* Check the front knee is over your ankle, not your toe. Also check the knee is not rolling in — if you draw an imaginary line down your knee cap and through to your foot it should be in line with your second toe. Don't be afraid to use a chair for extra balance. It's much better to perform the exercise with good technique.

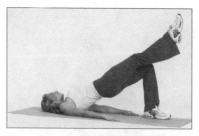

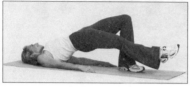

Body bit: Buttocks

The exercise: Ab bridge with leg lift

What it does: Tightens buttocks, strengthens pelvic stabilizers

Extra Body bit solution: Flattens abdominals and helps strengthen deep core trunk muscles important to your posture

Lie on your back your knees bent at 90 degrees and your feet under your knees. Contracting the abdominals, tilt the pelvis as you peel off the floor raising the body onto the shoulders, pushing your hips high. Keep the hips level and abdominals contracted to support the spine. Lift one leg straight and lift and lower it to the floor four times, contracting your buttocks as you lift. Take both feet flat to the floor and repeat on the other side.

> Joanna's top tip: This is a challenging exercise; make sure you do not drop the hips as you lift the leg. Pressing the knees away from your head will help you.

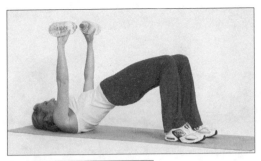

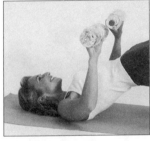

Body bit: Chest

The exercise: Ab Bridge with chest press

What it does: Shapes shoulders and pectorals

Extra Body bit solution: Tightens gluteals and hamstrings

Lying on your back with knees bent and feet flat on the floor, hold a dumbbell (or a 1–1.5 litre bottle of water) in each hand, with elbows bent at shoulder level. Tighten your buttocks and abdominals as you lift your buttocks off the floor into a bridge position. With the hips raised, press water bottles up over chest and then lower to start position. Maintain bridge and repeat chest press.

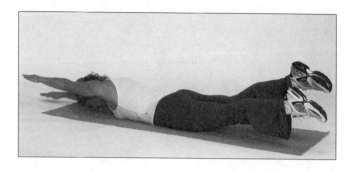

Body bit: Back

The exercise: Swimming

What it does: Tones the back muscles

Extra Body bit solution: Streamlines buttocks, thighs and arms

Lie face down on the floor with your abdominals contracted. Lift up your arms and legs and kick your arms and legs as if swimming. Keep the body lengthened as you do this and the head in line with the spine.

> Joanna's top tip: Imagine you are trying to reach something with your feet and fingertips. Start slowly with this exercise until you have perfected the technique.

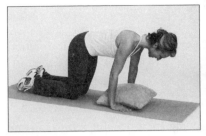 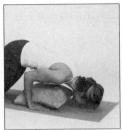

Body bit: Arms

The exercise: Cushion press up

What it does: Targets backs of arms

Extra Body bit solution: Deep stabilization of the abdominals means you get a tummy workout as well

Come into a box position, wrists under shoulders and knees under hips. Place a cushion between your hands with your hands positioned mid-way at the side of the cushion. Draw your elbows back so they are by your sides. Draw your body forward so your face is over the front of the cushion. Slowly lower your upper body down to the floor with your nose in front of the cushion. You will feel a tightening of the back of the arms. Keep the elbows tucked in as you push back up through your hands.

> _Joanna's top tip_: This may look easy but positioning the cushion means you can't cheat – check you keep your neck long and avoid hunching your ears down by your shoulders as you perform this exercise.

COOLING DOWN

Don't forget to cool down after each Total Body Solution workout. For ease, you can repeat your warm-up in reverse, decreasing the size of your movements and then finish off with the stretches below. Each stretch position is multi-functional, lengthening and stretching more than one body part. Hold each stretch position for 10–30 seconds.

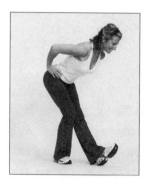

Exercise: Standing leg stretch

Stretches: Calves and hamstrings

Stand with good posture. Extend one leg in front of you, flexing the foot at the ankle. Bend the back knee and flex forward from the hips, contracting your abdominals as you extend forward. Lift up from the hips, checking they are level. Imagine you are balancing two glasses of water on each side of your lower back to help you. To progress the stretch, lift your leg and rest it on a bench, low step or chair.

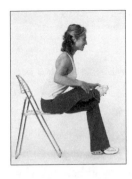

Exercise: Seated buttock stretch

Stretches: Buttocks and chest

Sit on a chair with good posture. Cross one ankle and rest on the other knee. Lean forward from the hips, extending tall through your spine, until you feel a stetch on your buttocks and outer hip. Draw your shoulders back to open and stretch the chest. To progress the stretch you can bring your weight onto your elbows and you should feel a deep stretch on the buttock of the crossed leg and across your chest.

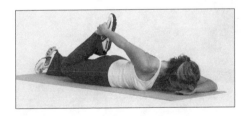

Exercise: Lying quad stretch

Stretches: Front thigh and hip flexor

Lie face down on the floor. Contract your abdominals to support your spine. Lift one leg into your bottom and reach back with the same hand as the lifted leg to hold onto the ankle or shoelaces. Keep the knees together and press the hips into the floor to increase the stretch.

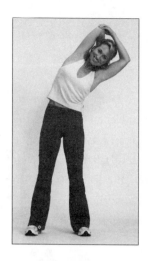

Exercise: Side stretch with triceps

Stretches: Waist muscles and back of arms.

Standing with good posture, extend one arm over your head and drop the hand between your shoulder blades. Support it with the other hand as you lean away from the elevated arm.

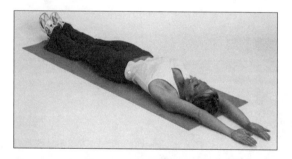

Exercise: Lying full body stretch

Stretches: Abdominals, thighs and shoulders

Lie on the floor face up. Extend your arms above your head. Gently stretch and lengthen through the whole body from your fingertips to your toes. Your lower back may come gently off the floor. Breathe gently and hold for up to 30 seconds. Slowly bring your arms down by your side.

HABIT 4

BE ORGANIZED – PLAN AHEAD

This strategy is all about being prepared. Prior preparation prevents poor performance – so the saying goes, and there is a lot of truth to it. If, for example, you had decided to start the *Get a Grip* plan and only read the instructions on Monday morning, you may well have decided not to bother, as you didn't have the right foods in the house, hadn't got time to fit in a walk, hadn't prepared any soup, and so on. You'd be far more likely to get off on the right foot if you had read the information through a few days before and got prepared. The same goes for exercise. A study on marathon runners in Japan found that those who dropped out during the race were those who had prepared least in training!

Developing the 'being prepared' habit focuses on two areas: being prepared with your food and exercise, and being prepared to deal with temptation.

PUTTING PLANNING INTO PRACTICE

PLAN YOUR MEALS

No one wants to come in from a busy day and spend hours in the kitchen. Having an idea of what you are going to cook is important in ensuring you have the necessary ingredients, and also being pre-warned of time needed for marinading, chopping and so on. For those days when time really is at a premium, check out our *On Your Plate in 15 minutes* recipes on page 225 for some really fast, easy and nutritious Starch Curfew supper ideas.

SHOPPING

If you are the sort of person who rushes to the shop on the way home to grab something for dinner, you may need to change your habits a little in order to achieve and maintain your weight loss goals. Why? Well, you're more likely to find yourself in the local takeaway if you've had a tiring day than buying things to cook if you never had a plan of what you were going to eat. Secondly, many late-opening shops have a poor selection of fresh vegetables and fruits. Writing a shopping list is essential – it will ensure you have what you need for the week ahead and it will also stop you wandering aimlessly up the aisles and being tempted by unhealthy food choices. Your shopping trolley should contain 40 per cent fruit and vegetables, but these don't all need to be fresh – frozen, canned and dried count too. OK you may need fresh veg for your salads, but think about frozen bags of fruit for smoothies, canned vegetables for adding to soups and stews, and frozen veg as accompaniments to your Starch Curfew suppers.

I'm a busy mum with a part-time job and feeding Jamie and Charlotte was always a rush – it just seemed so much easier to give them beans and sausages and have supper with them. I thought because I was having oven chips instead of deep-frying them, I was doing myself a real favour! I never thought I had the time to shop and cook healthily. Now I buy bags of pre-cut fresh and frozen veg, cooked chicken pieces and throw them all together in a stir-fry – it can be on the table in 10 minutes. I've even got into the habit of cooking a bit of extra rice to use the following day for my lunch – I add it to my soups or make a salad and take it to work. I've saved time and money and kept my weight off for 12 months – a total of 28 pounds.   **Emmaline, 28**

DELIVER ME FROM TEMPTATION!

Being prepared is not just about having the right foods on hand to help you select better choices. It is also about understanding how your body responds to temptation and the challenges you will come across. It's actually far easier to 'beat' temptation if you are expecting it. Think about this: when is your willpower strongest to avoid temptation? Chances are, it will be at the start of the day – you may not necessarily be a morning person but most people tend to find it easier to make healthier decisions in the morning. 'I'll opt for cereal and fruit for breakfast, rather than a Danish pastry at the work canteen' for example. As the day progresses and your energy levels start to flag, your willpower may start to dwindle, too, to the point that you can no longer resist the call of the vending machine by 4 p.m. If this is particularly pertinent to you, you may find the *Damage Limitation* section particularly helpful.

The brain is one of the most energy-demanding parts

of the body. It requires a constant flow of energy in the form of blood sugar. When our blood sugar drops too low, our ability to concentrate is directly affected and our willpower is greatly challenged. Maintaining stable blood sugar levels can help you sustain willpower. To achieve this, you need do three things:

1. Operate the Starch Curfew (see page 108)
2. Boost your intake of slow-releasing carbohydrates (see page 110)
3. Focus on your food ratios, especially at lunchtime (see number 8 page 157)
4. Keep well hydrated (see page 144)

TAKING ON TEMPTATION

CREATE DISTANCE

If you can't resist the urge to dig into the children's biscuit tin, then you need to create some distance between yourself and the tin. By distance, I mean not just putting the tin out of sight but creating a 'time distance' as well, to give you a little more time to get your willpower to kick in. Rather than telling yourself 'No, I can't have a biscuit,' say to yourself 'If I still really want one by the time I have taken those clothes upstairs and got the washing out the machine, then I'll reconsider.' By then, you may have summoned enough willpower to forgo the biscuit tin or, even better, you may have forgotten about it altogether!

I knew I had a problem with the kids' biscuit tin, so after trying many tricks to deny myself, I decided to put the tin in the cupboard with the ironing board and all the ironing. I knew I would have to face the task of doing the ironing every time I went to the cupboard for a biscuit. The strategy worked! Some days I don't even open the cupboard door as I don't want to look at the ironing and on other days I open the door intending to have a biscuit and my willpower kicks in – instead of digging into the biscuits I plough into my husbands shirts! On other days I set myself a target of ironing five shirts, taking them up and down the stairs and then allowing myself a biscuit. By the time I get that done – I often find the urge has gone. **Penny, 48**

RATE YOUR HUNGER

When hunger appears to strike, ask yourself if you are really hungry, or if you are actually bored, or thirsty, or just plain putting off a job you don't really want to do. If you can genuinely say you are hungry, then fine – have something to eat, prepare it and sit down to eat it. This is a far healthier strategy than simply popping food in your mouth and then being racked with guilt 20 minutes later when you realize you didn't really want it.

If, when you do start to eat, you find yourself overeating and unable to stop, try 'rating your hunger'. This is a really clever little trick. Before you eat, rate how hungry you are: 0 means you are starving while 5 means you are absolutely stuffed. Choose which number most closely represents how you feel. Studies have shown individuals who wait until their hunger rating is 0 before they eat actually take in more calories and are more likely to eat to a hunger rating of 5 (overeat) than individuals who sit down to eat when their hunger rating is 2.

So try to eat when you have a hunger rating of 2, but stop when you have a hunger rating of 4. As my grandfather used to say to my mum, you should always leave the table feeling you can eat just a little bit more.

LEARN TO SELF-TALK

This strategy is all about being prepared to give yourself a good talking to! When that little voice tries to lure you away from your good intentions, you need to be able to rationalize temptation and muster up willpower. For example, you set the alarm 10 minutes early, intending to go for a 10-minute power walk before you shower and go to work. But the alarm goes off and you think – I'll have the extra 10 minutes in bed and walk later. This is where developing self-talk is important. The following example illustrates how you can develop self-talk for yourself:

The alarm goes off …

You: I think I'll exercise later and have the extra snooze.
Self-talk: No, get up now and do it now – you know your day will get busy later on.
You: But I'm tired! I need the extra sleep.
Self-talk: An extra 10 minutes will not get rid of your

tiredness and besides, getting active is a great way to energize yourself.

You: But I'll do it later, after work.

Self-talk: You know that last time you did that, your day got too busy and your willpower was low, so you never did it. You might as well get up and do it now!

This is a simple scenario but developing self-talk through rationalization will help you be prepared and overcome the temptation to duck out of your good intentions.

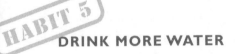

DRINK MORE WATER

Almost two-thirds of our body weight consists of it, every single cell is bathed in it and every single process in our bodies requires its presence. What is it? Water. And yet this vital nutrient is the one we most often overlook. If you rarely drink water, and instead quench thirst with tea, coffee or colas, you are probably in a constant state of dehydration. Not only does this prevent your body functioning optimally, it can also hamper your weight loss efforts, as fat can only be broken down in the presence of water. Study findings estimate that 30–40 per cent of us are mildly to moderately dehydrated. Research from the United States suggests we need 1ml of fluid per calorie of energy we consume. So if your average daily intake is 1600 calories, you need a minimum of 1.6 litres of water. While a balanced diet containing lots of fruit and veg can provide a proportion of this fluid, we should balance these sources with drinking water itself.

Adequate water consumption is even more important if you are a regular caffeine or alcohol drinker, as these substances both have a diuretic effect (meaning they cause your body to *lose* water). A study found that drinking six cups of coffee a day increased urinary excretion by 750ml – ¾ of a litre! A good rule of thumb is to consume one glass of water for every cup of caffeinated or alcoholic drink and to keep these to a minimum.

You may well have found that, initially, the water you drank during the 14-day plan had you in and out of the loo, but as your body becomes accustomed to consuming 2 litres of water a day, this will wear off. Hopefully, you're now significantly more active than you were before you started the plan – this too will have a bearing on how much water you need. If you are regularly active it is likely that you will need more than 2 litres of water a day to stay properly hydrated – we lose 500–1000ml of fluid per hour of exercise. A level of just 2 per cent dehydration will undermine your body's ability to perform exercise. To offset this loss, aim to drink 150ml–250ml every 15 minutes during a workout. Don't wait until you are thirsty – thirst is the body's last response to dehydration. Additionally, your brain can interpret thirst signals as hunger and this can cause unhealthy snacking. Your brain may be telling you to drink more water, but if you have got out of the habit, your brain will misinterpret this message as a need to eat more.

As you re-educate your thirst mechanism, you'll find it easier to understand what your body needs to keep your energy levels up.

One way of revealing how much water your body has lost during exercise is to weigh yourself before and after a vigorous exercise session. And yes, any change in your body weight is *solely* due to loss of fluid, as changes in fat and muscle composition don't come until later.

PUTTING THE WATER HABIT INTO PRACTICE

Much of the battle with adopting this strategy is simply getting used to it. It's not about denying yourself something or having to take time out to do something – it's simply about getting into the habit of remembering to drink it. Don't make the mistake of trying to drink a day's water allocation all at once. Not only is this not an effective way for you to maintain hydration, it will also make you feel bloated and uncomfortable, especially if you're about to do some exercise. Have a bottle of water on your desk at work, by the telephone at home and always carry a bottle in your bag.

When I first started the plan I couldn't imagine how I was ever going to be able to drink all that water. I felt like all I was doing was drinking water or going to the loo! I have always drunk lots of tea and coffee but I found that restricting my intake to two (or sometimes three) cups a day improved my energy levels and mood. I now carry a small bottle of water in my bag, always drink water with my meals and take a glass to bed with me every night. For someone who never touched the stuff a few weeks ago, that's pretty good going! **Joan, 63**

Devise a 'trigger' so that every time you do a particular thing (such as go to the loo, make a phone call or put the kettle on) you automatically drink a glass of water. If you're at work, aim to drink a glass for every hour that you are there − then you should be able to achieve the minimum 8 glasses a day.

WHICH WATER?

Any water is better than no water, regardless of whether it comes from a tap, a filter jug or a bottle. Sparkling water is not absorbed by the body tissues as quickly as still water, although it's fine to include some in your daily quota if you enjoy the taste. Experts also believe that water is best absorbed when drunk at room temperature rather than straight from the fridge. Research shows that the number one reason people fail to drink enough water is the taste − or lack of taste. Add a squeeze of lime or lemon, or infuse a slice of fresh ginger if you think water tastes too dull on its own. And drinking water is important for children too! Studies have shown that orange and grape flavours can be the most effective for stimulating a child to drink.

INCREASE YOUR INTAKE OF LIQUID FOODS

As you may have noticed, the 14-day plan included a high proportion of liquid-based foods, such as soups, juices and smoothies as well as water-based veg and fruit. This is a strategy well worth maintaining. Not only does it ensure you consume a large variety and volume of vitamin-packed fruits and vegetables, it can also assist your weight loss efforts.

TAKE YOUR FILL

You may well have found that the daily soup before your evening meal helped you feel full – especially in the absence of starchy accompaniments to your dinner. Well, if so, it's no surprise, as research from Penn State University found that foods with a high water content help stave off hunger. In the study, women who were served a soup prior to their meal ate fewer calories than those who were served a drier starter along with a glass of water.

The same team of researchers found that basing meals on water-packed foods enabled dieters to stick to a diet plan without feeling deprived or feeling that they had had to cut portion sizes dramatically. It makes sense: picture a sandwich filled with ham and a scrape of mustard. Now picture a sandwich containing a slice of ham and water-packed veg such as rocket leaves, tomato, onion and beetroot. It's easy to imagine which would leave you feeling more satisfied, not just physically but mentally, too.

We've already talked about the importance of water consumption as part of a healthy lifestyle, but water shouldn't replace liquid-based foods as a weight loss strategy – the Penn State researchers found that drinking water with meals wasn't effective in reducing calorie intake.

Oh, and a word of warning – liquid based foods doesn't mean liquid lunches! A study in the *American Journal of Clinical Nutrition* found that just a single pre-lunch wine or beer resulted in less post-meal satiety and increased calorie intake over the next 24 hours.

PUTTING THE LIQUID FOODS STRATEGY INTO PRACTICE

First and foremost, don't drop the juices and soups from your daily diet – even if you're not hungry – and make sure you include fruits and vegetables from the suggested lists to accompany your meals. The varieties selected are particularly high in water, so they'll make you feel fuller than other types.

The mid-morning juice and pre-dinner soup definitely helped me to stick with the plan. Just as hunger began to strike, I'd remember to have my juice and then I'd feel able to carry on until lunchtime. The soup ensures you don't feel deprived at dinnertime and, for me, that was really important as I was wondering how I would ever cope with potato- or rice-free meals! **Sam, 33**

If you're pushed for time, prepare the fruit or veg you need for the juices in the morning so you can just throw them in the juicer or blender when you want them. Or fall back on a shop-bought option. When you make a soup, do a job lot and freeze what you don't need for the next few days. For variety, make a couple of different recipes and freeze them in small boxes so that you don't have to have the same one every night. Check out the recipe section in the appendices for more tasty, filling soup and smoothie recipes.

Another easy way to include more liquid-based foods in your daily diet is by checking out the incredibly simple liquid-based meal options in the table overleaf. These can work as starch curfew soups and stews or filling lunches, depending on when you choose to eat them. If it's for lunch, add half a cup of cooked pasta or brown rice to your soup as it cooks, 2 chopped boiled potatoes or 2 tablespoons of barley. Alternatively, serve with a wholemeal brown roll. They are all quick to make, nutritious and versatile. Enjoy!

QUICK AND EASY LIQUID MEALS

This is so simple – all you do is:

1. Take a soup base
2. Add a protein option
3. Chuck in a vegetable option, eat and enjoy!

Follow the ideas overleaf or make up your own quick and easy liquid meals.

Soup base	Protein option	Vegetable option	What you do
Tomato and Basil	Cottage cheese	Chopped tomatoes and fresh basil	Heat the soup, add the chopped tomatoes and heat through. Pour into a bowl, top with the cottage cheese and sprinkle with the fresh basil.
Carrot and Coriander	Canned chickpeas	Leeks, carrots and onions	In a non-stick pan, soften the chopped onion, carrot and leeks. When soft, add the soup and drained chickpeas. Heat thoroughly and serve. Feeling posh? Garnish with a tablespoon of yoghurt and sprinkle of cumin.
Chilled cucumber	Canned salmon	Cucumber and broccoli	Heat the soup, add the chopped cucumber and broccoli and cook until the vegetables are *al dente*. Add the drained salmon and heat through. Feeling posh? Serve with chopped cucumber on top with a drizzle of Thai sweet chilli sauce.

Soup base	Protein option	Vegetable option	What you do
Chicken and sweetcorn	Chicken breast	Mange tout, canned or fresh sweetcorn	In a non-stick pan, soften the mange tout and sweet-corn over a moderate heat. Add the chicken breast and stir. Heat thoroughly and serve. Add a little soy sauce to the mange tout and chicken while heating for a bit of a Chinese flavour.
Tomato, red pepper and lime	Mixed seafood (mussels, prawns, calamari, cockles)	Onion and red pepper	In a non-stick pan, soften the chopped onion and red pepper over a moderate heat. Stir in a tablespoon of Thai sweet chilli sauce. Add the seafood and heat thoroughly. Stir in the soup and heat through.
Tomato	Canned tuna	Watercress and cucumber	Chop the watercress and steam with the cucumber in a little water. Add the soup and drained tuna and heat thoroughly. Serve with a dollop of natural yoghurt.

Soup base	Protein option	Vegetable option	What you do
Mushroom	Cold roast lean beef	Mushrooms – different types work particularly well	In a non-stick pan, soften the mushrooms. Add the chopped meat and the soup and heat through. Serve with chopped raw mushrooms, or, for extra zing, you can saute the mushrooms in a little garlic and hot grainy mustard.
Gazpacho	Hard-boiled egg	Chopped red onion, red and yellow pepper and cucumber	Pour the soup into a bowl, garnish with the chopped vegetables and top with the chopped boiled egg.

With the exception of the Gazpacho, remember to heat all the soups thoroughly before serving. Do not boil soups excessively, however, as this can damage the flavour.

HABIT 7

TIME YOUR EXERCISE TO SUIT YOU

In *Get a Grip*, we aimed to get you active as early in the day as possible. Not only does getting off on the right foot help you stick with the plan all day, evidence shows that people who exercise in the morning are more likely to stick with a long-term programme. It makes sense, as first thing, there are fewer obstacles to get between you and your workout. We also spread bouts of activity throughout the day, as these are often easier to fit in than one extended exercise session.

If, after the two-week plan, you still find 'early bird' exercise a pain, worry not! Research on performance and time of day suggests that we can work *harder* without perceiving it to be so in the late afternoon to early evening. A study from the University of North Texas found that volunteers were able to work 26 per cent harder in the afternoon than in the morning, which perhaps helps suggest why most Olympic records have been set in the late afternoon and early evening. Other research shows that our body's aerobic system responds to exercise more quickly in the afternoon compared to the morning. As far as how often you exercise during the day goes, some research suggests that the effect on metabolism of repeated bouts of exercise is greater than when you restrict physical activity to just one daily slot. If you are continuing to exercise in small bouts, aim to keep them to 15–20 minutes. A study found that 5–10 minute bouts, whilst having a beneficial effect on metabolism, did not have such a strong impact on blood lipids (fats). The overall message is to do what works for you. If your body tells you that exercise is easier and more enjoyable in the evening, then plan your day to include a later workout. If you'd rather grab 10 minutes every few hours than put aside a whole hour, fine. Fit in exercise where you can. The fact that you're doing it is far more important than time of day.

PUTTING SUITABLE TIMING INTO PRACTICE

Experiment with exercise at different times of day. You may surprise yourself by finding you love the peace and quiet of the early morning for a power walk or enjoy winding down with a late evening yoga class. Contrary to popular belief, light exercise before bedtime doesn't keep you awake – in fact, one study found that it helped subjects get off to the land of Nod more quickly and enhanced the quality of their sleep.

Listen to your body – if you need to go more gently in the morning (research shows that it takes us longer to get going in the morning as we age) then do so. Muscles and joints are at their stiffest early on, too, so make sure you're thoroughly warmed up before stretching. As far as muscles go, experts say that strength peaks in the afternoon to early evening. Why not try the Total Body Solution workout (page 120) in this time slot and see if it feels easier.

Do what you can, when you can – it may end up being all you do if the trials and tribulations of the day get in the way. If you don't seize an exercise opportunity when you can, you may miss out altogether. While it is often recommended that you try to spread your exercise sessions throughout the week, it won't make much difference in physical terms. Studies do show, however, that people tend to feel they've achieved more when they are able to spread exercise evenly throughout the week.

Although I am not what you'd call a morning person, I made the effort to get up and do the pre-breakfast walk and abdominal exercises. This helped me to remain positive throughout the 14 days as if work got really busy and stressful and prevented me from doing any more walking, I knew that I'd at least done something.   **Sam, 33**

HABIT 8

FIGURE OUT YOUR FOODS

It's fairly obvious that in order to lose weight and body fat, you need to use more calories than you are consuming. This needs to be achieved through a combination of sensible nutrition and physical exercise. To reduce body fat you need to create a deficit of 3500 calories a week. This figure can appear alarming, but don't panic! The secret to effective weight and body fat loss is to ensure that the calorie burn is achieved slowly and consistently. Spreading the 3500 calories over seven days means you are aiming for a decrease of 500 calories each day. If you split these 500 calories between physical activity, structured exercise and nutritional habit grooving, it becomes a lot more manageable. You do not need to put your life on hold to reach your healthy weight and body fat goals.

GETTING THE BALANCE RIGHT

Many people experience changes in their energy levels when they start a 'diet'. Feelings of tiredness can relate to the fact that the body is having to survive on fewer calories than it is used to. Nutritional Habit Grooving is not about getting you to continually survive on fewer and fewer calories, but about learning to apply techniques that help you match your energy intake with the amount of energy you need. In this section, I'll explain how you can figure out your foods in relation to the different properties and calorie values of the main nutrient groups – and why you need the right balance of all three. If you look back at *Get a Grip*, you'll see many of the volunteers commented on how much more energy they had. This in part relates to the fact that they were eating the right nutrients in the right ratios at the right time.

WHERE DOES ENERGY COME FROM?

The main food groups – proteins, fats and carbohydrates – provide the body with energy. The body uses this energy to carry out its everyday activities, from going to pick up the kids from school, completing structured exercise and even digesting your food. Energy is measured in calories, but not all foods give the same amount of energy. You'll see from the table below that one gram of fat provides nearly twice the amount of energy as one gram of protein. (Alcohol also provides the body with energy – 7 Kcals per gram – but it is not a nutrient as it is not necessary for life.)

Nutrient	Energy per gramme Kcals
Carbohydrate	4
Fat	9
Protein	4

The amount of calories you are eating is important, but it is not the whole story when it comes to sustaining a healthy diet – different foods, and combinations of foods, affect the rate at which your body receives energy and even affect the brain differently. This is a fascinating area, and once you have learned to balance your food intake, you will really notice a huge difference in your ability to concentrate and maintain motivation.

You learned about the Glycaemic Index in section two, so you know that some foods produce a sharp rise in blood sugar and a subsequent dip in energy, often accompanied by cravings for more starchy foods. But did you know that many starch-rich foods such as bread, pasta, rice and potatoes increase the amount of serotonin your body produces? This brain transmitter has a 'calming' effect, and can cause feelings of lethargy. If you have ever experienced that post-lunch slump – a feeling of wanting to put your head down on your desk or eat a chunk of chocolate to give you 'energy' to get through the afternoon (even though you have just had your lunch!) – you may be getting your food ratios wrong.

Starch-based foods do provide us with an important energy source, but the trick is to get the balance right, and this is where food ratios come in.

It is a really simple concept that involves eating an equal amount of protein with your starch. This slows down the release of blood sugar, dampens the effect of serotonin and helps maintain your energy levels.

Ideally, your lunchtime meal should include an equal amount of protein and starch – that means a ratio of one to one. You don't need to weigh things out to achieve this – you can simply estimate it by what the foods look like. Take a ham sandwich as an example. The sandwich has two slices of bread (the starch) and a slice of ham (protein);

the ratio is therefore two to one. To get a better ratio, ditch the top slice of bread and add a slice more ham so it looks about the same quantity as the slice of bread. Now add a side salad or pile on a bag of salad with chopped tomatoes and peppers and you have got yourself a perfect one to one food ratio lunch. The great thing about food ratios is that it works for everyone: the whole family can benefit even if they do not want to lose weight – all you have to do is give them an equal amount of starch and protein at lunch.

Starch isn't the only energy-influencing nutrient. Protein-rich foods such as chicken, tofu, fish, lean red meat and pulses stimulate the release of dopamine in the brain, which increases our ability to concentrate and focus. Make sure you get sufficient protein in your diet, whether it is from meat and fish sources or pulses and vegetables. It is important for everyone to have a varied diet of fruit and vegetables, as eating too much protein decreases the body's ability to absorb vitamin C and vitamin B. Absorption of these two vitamins is especially suppressed if you suffer from stress. In these situations, the body actually produces more homocysteine, a compound that has been implicated in an increased risk of heart disease. Eating a diet rich in fruit and vegetables will help you increase your intake of vitamins C and B and readdress the balance – another reason why the Starch Curfew is beneficial to your health!

FIGURING OUT FATS

As you can see from the table above, the fat in our food is the most concentrated source of energy (calories). But this is not to say we should be cutting out all fat in the diet. Nearly all of us need to decrease our fat intake, but it is not a case of having no fat. Some fat is important for normal health – it protects organs like the liver and kidneys, it plays a role in enabling and sustaining pregnancy and it helps keep us warm. Some vitamins – A, D, E and K – are 'fat-soluble', meaning that fat must be present in order for them to be broken down and used by the body. Some foods contain essential fats, which our bodies cannot make themselves. In addition, research has shown an association between depression and very low fat diets.

So how much is enough? Ideally, total fat intake should provide no more than 30 per cent of the total calories in our diet. This means that if your calorie intake falls within the recommended female daily requirements of 1900–2100 calories per day, then you should be consuming no more than 63–72 grams of fat per day. For a male, the recommended daily requirements are 2100–2500 calories per day, allowing 70–83 grams of fat per day. A study of 2200 British adults found that the average intake of fat for women was 74 grams, and for men, 102 grams per day. Check out the table below to see how replacing a fattening favourite with a healthy alternative a few times a week can make a difference to your weight …

Fattening Favourite	Tasty Alternative	Calories saved if you swap your fattening fave for your tasty alternative twice a week	Over the course of a year, you'll save yourself ... (remember, 3500 calories = 1lb of fat!)	Potential weight loss over 1 year
Chunk of cheese (1oz) 115 Kcals	Half-fat Cheddar 75 Kcals	80 Kcals	4160 Kcals	1.2lbs
1 chocolate digestive 85 Kcals	1 rough oatcake 55 Kcals	60 Kcals	3120 Kcals	0.9lbs
Large handful of tortilla chips (50g) 245 Kcals	Large handful of plain popcorn (28g) 165 Kcals	160 Kcals	8320 Kcals	2.4lbs
Rich and creamy rice pudding (½ can) 190 Kcals	Canned peaches with small pot of fruit yoghurt 90 Kcals	200 Kcals	10,400 Kcals	3lbs
1 prawn and egg deep-filled sandwich 570 Kcals	Boots Shapers prawn, lemon and chilli mayo sandwich, 265 Kcals	710 Kcals	36,920 Kcals	10.5lbs
½ pot taramasalata 400 Kcals	½ pot reduced fat houmous 210 Kcals	380 Kcals	19,760 Kcals	5.6lbs

For weight management purposes, I recommend a daily fat intake of 30–40 grams. However, all fats are not created equal and in your efforts to reduce fat intake it is best to focus on specific types of fat. These include saturated and trans fat sources. Other types of fats, such as essential fatty acids found in oily fish, should be maintained or even increased. For health purposes, fat intake should never fall below 10 grams a day.

FIGURE OUT YOUR FATS

Check out the table opposite to learn more about the different types of fat in our diet and which ones to approach with caution.

Note: The polyunsaturated essential fatty acids – omega-6 and omega-3 – are considered 'essential' because our bodies are unable to manufacture them. They must therefore be obtained from our diet.

ALWAYS READ THE LABEL

Food labels can be very misleading. For example, peanut butter labels may read 'cholesterol free' – this is true, but the peanut butter never had cholesterol in it in the first place! And cholesterol free does *not* mean fat free. Some cereal manufacturers claim 'no added fat' on muesli or wholesome cereal products, yet the natural grains have been processed with coconut or palm oils, which are high in saturated fat. One food may be described on the label as 'low fat' but in actual fact this may be a relative

Fat Type	Typical Sources	Health Effect	Recommendations
Saturated Fat	Meat, dairy products and some tropical oils including palm oil and cocoa butter	Increases cholestrol levels. Increases risk of heart disease and certain cancers	The less the better. No more than 10% of total calories. (In a 1000-Kcal diet that would be 10g – equivalent to 2 tsps!)
Trans Fatty Acids – mostly man-made molecules produced during hydrogenation of vegetable oil, a process used in the manufacture of various foodstuffs including margarine	Margarine, shortening, fried foods, breads, crackers, snack foods, spreads, processed/prepared foods	Has a negative effect on cholesterol – decreases the HDL (good) and increases the LDL (bad). May increase risk of heart disease and breast cancer	The less the better, minimize consumption. Avoid products that use the words 'hydrogenated' or 'partially hydrogenated' on the label
Monounsaturated Fatty Acids	Olive, rapeseed, almond, cashew, hazelnut, macadamia, pecan and peanut oils	Has a beneficial effect on cholesterol levels. Lowers LDL and maintains HDL	Olive oil and rapeseed oil are the best choices. Should make up 12% of total calories

Fat Type	Typical Sources	Health Effect	Recommendations
POLYUNSATURATED FATS			
Omega-6 Essential Fatty Acids	Corn, safflower, sesame, soybean, sunflower oils, nuts and wheatgerm	Consuming too many of these vegetable oils can alter the delicate balance of omega-6 and omega-3 fats	Limit consumption of these vegetable oils – should make up no more than 10% of total calories. Avoid heating these delicate oils – instead use olive oil or rapeseed oil for cooking
Omega-3 Essential Fatty Acids	Cold-water fish (salmon, mackerel, herring, halibut, tuna and sardines). Flaxseed, hempseed, walnuts and their oils, soybean oils, green leafy vegetables	Inhibits blood clots, reduces risk of heart disease, increases immune function	Increase consumption to 3–6g daily. (Have oily fish 3 times a week or 1 tsp freshly ground flaxseed daily)

term comparing what is essentially a high fat food to the even higher fat standard product. Mayonnaise is a classic example of this – even the 'low fat' version can hardly be described as low in calories.

The information on food labels can help you compare the types and amount of fat in specific foods.

Here are some quick guidelines to look for:

1. Look at total fat intake and not just saturated fat. Any fat, healthy or not, provides 9 calories per gram.
2. Just because it says 'low fat' on the front does not necessarily mean it is a low-fat food. An apple is a naturally low-fat food while 'low-fat' mayo is not!
3. Avoid trans fats by looking for the term 'hydrogenated'. The higher up the list you see this term, the more hydrogenated unhealthy fats are in the food.
4. It may say reduced fat on the label but do check out the total calories – the extra flavour may be added through the use of extra sugars and processed flavourings.

HABIT 9

EXERCISE PORTION CONTROL

Few people know what a 'standard' portion looks like. In experiments in which people are asked to prepare a standard-sized meal, the vast majority cook up portions

2–3 times the size recommended by government health guidelines. It's not really surprising – eat out at a restaurant or buy a takeaway and you'll frequently be served a meal big enough for two or three people. A coffee boutique 'tall' coffee can contain three times the amount of caffeine of a standard cup. A study in the *American Journal of Public Health* recently found that in the States, portion sizes are 2–5 times bigger than they were 30 years ago – and judging from the burgeoning problem with obesity, the people who are eating them are too! The amount you eat is important, regardless of what the food is. Take white bread, for example – a basic foodstuff in most people's kitchen containing no fat. Yet if you eat enough of it, you'll gain weight. The same goes for apples, chicken breasts, porridge – you name it. The fact is we have to exercise portion control in order to achieve weight control.

Since completing the 14-day plan, you probably have a far better idea of portion sizes. To help you maintain a visual picture of what a standard portion of a particular food looks like – so that you don't get led astray by gigantic restaurant or takeaway shop portions – we've included a reference list of food portions sized by everyday household objects.

PORTION SIZES IN THE REAL WORLD

Cheese – a matchbox-sized piece (30g/1oz) equals one serving

Rice – your fist equates to about a cup, a standard portion of rice should be ½ cup (uncooked)

Pasta – a helping the size of your computer mouse when uncooked

Fish – a piece the size of a woman's palm (85g/3oz) equals one serving

Meat or poultry – a piece the size of a credit card, about 2.5cm/½ inch thick (85g/3oz) equals one serving

1 bagel – the size of a compact disc

1 slice of pizza – should be no bigger than a standard white business envelope

When I started the plan and prepared some of the recipes included, I was amazed at how small the portions appeared to be. It would say 'serves 4' when I'd think there was just about enough for two! Yet, once supplemented with a juicy salad or some tasty vegetables I found the meals recommended to be perfectly satisfying. I realized then how big the helpings I'd been eating before were. **Sam, 33**

PUTTING PORTION CONTROL INTO PRACTICE

- Get into the habit of weighing foods to see how much constitutes a single serving. You won't need to do it forever, as you'll soon be familiar enough with the amounts to simply estimate them.
- When you've prepared and served your recommended helping size of a particular meal, put the remainder away immediately.

If you leave the bowl on the table or the bread on the bread-board you'll be tempted to have a little bit extra.

■ Serve your meal on a smaller plate so that it fills it up. No matter how appetizing it smells, a small meal on a vast white plate isn't the most appealing prospect.

HABIT 10

EAT PLENTY OF FIBRE

The high intake of fruit and vegetables in the *Get a Grip* plan ensured that your intake of fibre was high. Studies show that foods rich in fibre tend to be more bulky and less calorie-dense than low-fibre foods. They take longer to chew and they slow the rate of digestion (and therefore blood sugar release) down, enabling you to feel fuller for longer. The result? You are less likely to overeat. Research from Penn State University in the United States found that fibre was one of the key secrets in feeling satiated while reducing calorie intake. There are other benefits to be gained, too. In a study of 139 people, those who started eating cereal packed with 6–12g of fibre daily reported feeling more energetic than those who began the day with a low-fibre cereal. Asked to rate their energy levels, the high-fibre crowd gave themselves scores 10 per cent higher than the low-fibre-eating group. They also reported feeling better and thinking more clearly.

Why? Most likely, at least in part, by alleviating that

common little problem that no one likes to talk about: con-stipation. Studies report that individuals who switch to high-fibre diets feel more energetic because they feel lighter and more comfortable. The average diet contains around 13g of fibre or less a day. This has been associated with stool weights of less than 100g a day, which, in turn, have been linked to a raised risk of bowel disease. Eating more fibre can also help lower the risk of diabetes, heart disease, and possi-bly cancer, and can help control your weight. In addition, soluble fibre, such as that found in porridge oats and pulses, is thought to have a beneficial effect on cholesterol levels.

HOW MUCH FIBRE DO I NEED?

You should be getting 18–32g a day. Increasing your fibre intake to 18g a day translates into a 25 per cent increase in stool weight. It might not sound like a very attractive prospect, but it will make you feel healthier and more ener-getic. You may find it takes your system a few days to adjust to a higher fibre intake, but stay with it. In the study mentioned above, the high-fibre group did experience more abdominal bloating at first but this eased during the second week.

PUTTING FIBRE ON THE MENU

Getting more fibre in your diet doesn't mean eating bowlfuls of bran and munching on celery sticks all day long. You can increase fibre intake by making a few small changes to your shopping and eating habits. Here are a few ideas:

- Opt for wholemeal flour instead of white flour in baking and choose wholemeal bread instead of white, most of the time.
- Use wholemeal varieties of rice and pasta. Wholemeal pasta has 3.5 grams of fibre per 100g compared to just 1.2 grams in white pasta.
- Serve every meal with a variety of vegetables or salad – scrape rather than peel or leave skins intact to retain the maximum amount of fibre.
- Ensure you eat at least 3 pieces of fruit a day – oranges are particularly high in fibre, as are berry fruits such as raspberries, and dried fruits and sultanas pack a fibre punch in a concentrated form.

Breakfast is an ideal opportunity to add more fibre to your diet. A single bowl of high-fibre cereal can narrow the deficit.

If you like ...	Switch to ...	Your Fibre Boost ...
Crunchy Nut cornflakes 0.9g	Bran flakes 4.2g	3.3g
Special K 0.8g	Fruit 'n' Fibre 2.7g	1.9g
Ready Brek 2.7g	2 Weetabix 4.4g	1.7g
Rice Krispies 0.5g	Shreddies 3.4g	2.9g

Hopefully, you have started to groove some of these habits already. Over the next few weeks and months, try to add in one more strategy to your weight loss efforts until they all become regular practice. Don't worry if some take longer to get the hang of than others, and don't beat yourself up if you go off the rails every now and then. Accept that accidents do occur, and simply get back to your new healthy lifestyle. In recognition of the fact that life isn't always what we would ideally like it to be, the next section, *Damage Limitation*, is devoted to crisis management. Read on to find out more …

Life may not always run smoothly so to keep your new size you need ...

DAMAGE LIMITATION

Have you noticed that as your weight loss dreams become a reality and exercise a regular part of your life, you start to get a feel-good factor – a kind of rush that actually makes you want to carry on eating sensibly and exercising? You actually reach a situation where you are enjoying your healthy lifestyle. As you get to grips with the strategies you learned about in section two, you begin to climb up a self-perpetuating spiral, you look and feel better, you have more energy, which spurs you on to continue.

There you are, looking great, feeling in control, with bags more energy, then BANG! Real life hits you with a genuine crisis or obstacle and your healthy lifestyle goes out the window – just when you felt you were doing so well.

So, you get thrown off your upward spiral and find yourself plunging back to where you started, making unhealthy food choices, having no motivation to exercise and, worst of all, feeling guilty and as if you have failed or let yourself down. You start to feel annoyed with yourself and a bit depressed, which prevents you from taking control of the situation. Eventually, you hit the bottom and if you're lucky, pick yourself up and start again.

THE SPIRAL SCENARIO

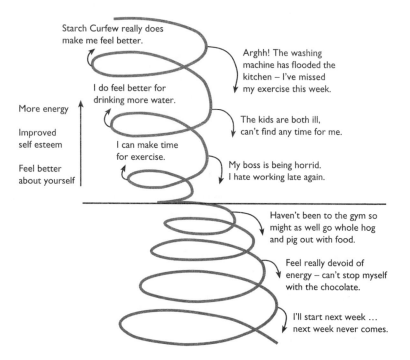

Starch Curfew really does make me feel better.

Arghh! The washing machine has flooded the kitchen – I've missed my exercise this week.

I do feel better for drinking more water.

The kids are both ill, can't find any time for me.

More energy

Improved self esteem

I can make time for exercise.

Feel better about yourself

My boss is being horrid. I hate working late again.

Haven't been to the gym so might as well go whole hog and pig out with food.

Feel really devoid of energy – can't stop myself with the chocolate.

I'll start next week … next week never comes.

These peaks and troughs of weight gain and weight loss and the accompanying psychological battle we have with ourselves can be damaging not only to our body's health but also to our long-term self-esteem and body image. Studies show that women with low self-esteem and negative body image are less likely to exercise and more likely to practise unhealthy eating behaviours such as fasting and bingeing or using laxatives and diet pills. So how can you avoid being thrown off your upward spiral? It is how you deal with life's rich and varied situations that can really make an impact on your long-term success. So instead of letting such difficulties get the better of you, in this section you'll find a variety of problems and solutions to help you keep on track. I call this Damage Limitation.

WHAT IS DAMAGE LIMITATION?

The key to practising successful damage limitation is learning how to identify and deal with potentially problematic situations. Sometimes, they are small things − like nibbling the childrens' leftovers − that have just become a habit that's really difficult to break, or maybe a bigger event − like a weekend of partying at a wedding, or a traditional Sunday lunch get-together − has you in a panic. Maybe you are a chocoholic, or stress has you reaching for the vending machine. Whatever it is, we all have a situation where we find self-control difficult, or even impossible, and we often find ourselves ditching all our good intentions. And you know what? That is OK − it is OK to have some chocolate, it is OK to have that splurge − life is about having a good time, after all. But the problem comes when we see one minor hiccup as the end of everything positive we have achieved. Yes, we all get knocked off our spiral every now and then but, instead of helter-skeltering all the way down, damage limitation will help you find solutions to the challenges and problems you experience in your life, enabling you to maintain weight loss, an active lifestyle and a healthy body image. Not all the following situations will present a challenge to you, but there are plenty of solutions, tips and recipes that you can incorporate into your own damage limitation strategy.

If you feel that maintaining a healthy diet and finding time to exercise is just too much, you may feel that you can only do one or the other. If you put me on the spot, I'd have to say that being physically active – whether it's through Moving More, More Often, or through Structured Exercise – is the single most important strategy you can adopt and maintain; it directly improves your health, helps boost your self-esteem and controls your body composition – meaning you will be burning more calories, even in your sleep. What you eat is of the utmost importance too, but if one is going to be temporarily put aside due to other commitments or difficulties, do try to keep up your physical activity.

PROBLEM:

THE FAMILY ALL EAT AT DIFFERENT TIMES

Not eating as a family can cultivate some bad eating habits, not just with you but also with the rest of the family. A week-long survey of 289 senior school children by the Childrens' Nutrition Research Center in Dallas revealed youngsters who had dinner with their parents ate lower fat foods and more fruit and vegetables. Overweight children reported eating at least half of their meals in front of the television. Meanwhile, a Spanish study of 282 teenagers who shared at least five family meals a week, found they suffered less anxiety and depression, regardless of their parents' education level or whether both parents worked outside of the home.

SOLUTION: DAMAGE LIMITATION

■ Make a family dinner date

Check schedules and make a date when you can sit down together for dinner. Mark everyone's calendars and tell them their attendance at dinner is requested. You could even write invites to make it more of a special occasion.

■ Bring home healthy, fast food

Try pre-cut, frozen, canned or microwave-in-the-bag veg. Turn up the nutrition on canned soups by adding frozen vegetables and pre–cooked chicken breasts.

■ Dig out the slow cooker

Toss in frozen chicken breasts, a bag of frozen carrots, chopped onions and a jar of low-salt sauce before you leave for work. Your meal will then be ready when you are.

■ Sit down on the run

If you only have time for a quick bite at a fast food outlet (see below) you can still make it a healthy affair. For example, choose grilled chicken with no sauce and remove the skin, or a single burger with lettuce and tomato instead of a triple cheeseburger. Order side salads (hold the dressing) and skip the fizzy drinks, opting instead for low-fat milk, water and juice. Unfortunately, pizza can be a nutritional minefield, laden with cheese, high-fat meat and oil. The main problem, however, is the size of the helping you're usually given. If you're eating out, share a pizza with a friend and fill up with a side salad. Or ask the restaurant to use half the usual amount of cheese along with a variety of vegetable toppings.

PROBLEM: EATING OUT

Let's get one thing straight – living a healthy, balanced life should be about going out and having a good time. Long-term weight management should not leave you feeling you cannot accept invitations from friends and family or enjoy a meal in a restaurant while you are grooving your new healthy eating habits. So when your dinner invitation arrives here are some solutions to help you.

SOLUTION: DAMAGE LIMITATION

■ Operate a starch-free zone

A starch-free zone is a useful strategy to help you keep

your calories balanced when operating the Starch Curfew just isn't possible. Instead of having a Starch Curfew dinner and causing all sorts of complications for your host, have a Starch Curfew lunch instead. This allows you to include some starch with your evening meal without over-indulging.

When eating out at a friends, I usually go along with whatever they are having rather than causing a fuss. But I do not have such big portions as I used to do, or go back for second helpings. I also skip the bread and stick to just one glass of wine. When eating out in a restaurant, I used to allow myself whatever I wanted – it wasn't until I started the plan and kept track of my eating habits that I realized how often I ate out and acknowledged that I needed to choose more suitable options. Whilst on holiday recently, out of four nights eating in restaurants, I had baked hake, grilled lemon sole, fillet steak and monkfish. No calorie-laden sauces, deep-frying or desserts for me! Changed times, thanks to the Get a Grip *plan.*
Joan, 63

■ Eat in two acts

This is a useful strategy for those of us who overeat when away from our home territory. Divide the food on your plate in two halves. If you are dining out you can make an imaginary line. Eat half the food. Stop for 10 minutes and either leave the table, or sip a glass of water until empty. If you are still hungry after 10 minutes, finish your meal. If you are not sure, divide the remainder in half and repeat the exercise.

■ Order first, drink later

Place your food order before you have your glass of wine. Alcohol loosens your inhibitions, which makes you less careful when ordering. It also makes you feel less satisfied after your meal, resulting in an increased calorie intake over the next 24 hours.

■ My usual, please

If you have a favourite restaurant that you visit frequently, decide ahead what you would like to order, basing your choice on the Habit Grooving principles you learned in Section Two. That way, you won't be tempted when you open the menu. When your resolve is weak, tell someone what you would like to order and visit the cloakroom while the order is being taken so your decision can't be shaken.

■ Buffet Management

Buffets are the dieter's downfall. An American study recently found that people ate a staggering 44 per cent more when they were able to select from a variety of dishes, compared to being offered the same amount of just one dish. So at buffets, try limiting your variety of foods to two per plate, that way you are not over-eating all in one go. Allow yourself to go back as many times as you wish but enjoy the flavours you have on your plate one at one time.

■ Portion Control

Fill your plate with vegetables, salad and lower calorie foods and then top off with one or two of the other buffet fillers, remembering to keep a check on portion sizes. Turn to page 166 for a reminder of what a standard portion of some common foods looks like.

■ Prioritize your eating

Once back at your table eat the lowest calorie foods first (these are generally the vegetables). Then eat the next lowest calorie item. Save your highest calorie item for last. You'll get the taste, but you may just find yourself too full to finish it.

■ Don't starve, eat less

If you know you've got a splurge coming, try eating a little less the day before. Aim to eat 300 calories less, make sure you meet your physical activity targets, and you can enjoy your excesses a little more without feeling guilty. The day after you overeat return to your habit grooving.

PROBLEM:

YOU ARE STRESSED

Stress is a very common trigger for overeating – you either do it to 'comfort' yourself from the trials and tribulations of the day, or you do it mindlessly – barely aware that you are eating at all. Just look at how this 'mindless nibbling' can impact on your weight loss efforts ...

THE PERILS OF MINDLESS NIBBLING

Food	What it costs in calories	If you did it every day you'd gain ...	If you were able to do it only twice a week you'd save ...
2 teaspoons peanut butter	125	13lbs in a year	625 kcals
Large handful of salted peanuts	300	31lbs in a year	1500 kcals
Tablespoon of cake mixture	120	12.5lbs in a year	600 kcals
Matchbox-sized piece of cheese	115	12lbs in a year	575 kcals
Finishing off kids' 2 sausages	220	23lbs in a year	1100 kcals
Eating the children's left-over buttered toast	130 a slice	13.5lbs in a year	650 kcals
Handful of fries	115 (for half a small bag)	12lbs in a year	575 kcals

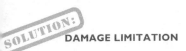

DAMAGE LIMITATION

■ Opt for 'eat slow' snacks

Foods that are hard to eat take longer to finish, which gives the brain a chance to register what you have actually put in your stomach. Here are some ideas: a baked apple, a large bowl of air-popped popcorn, a bag of pre-cut carrots with low-fat dip, or an artichoke with low-fat dressing.

■ Move more, more often

Exercise, particularly low to moderate intensity aerobic activity, has been shown to reduce stress and anxiety. Refer back to Move More, More Often and Structured Exercise on pages 102 and 116 for ideas on how to inject a little more activity into your life and combat stress.

■ Get a proper perspective

Acknowledging that you are in a stressful phase of your life is really important. Now is the time to praise yourself for any healthy activity or strategy you are maintaining, rather than beating yourself up for not doing more. So even if you've failed to operate the Starch Curfew or fit in structured exercise, perhaps you've managed to drink your daily quota of water and walked to the station every day. Be patient with yourself, and practise a positive mantra such as 'I am taking care of my body while it sees me through this stressful situation.'

■ Raise yourself up the priority list

Get a piece of paper and answer the following questions:
Who is the most important person in your life?
After that person, who is the most important person in your life?

Look at the names you wrote down. Do you see your name? If you do, well done. If you don't, think how many more layers of other 'more' important people you would list before you wrote down your own name. If you are the primary homemaker in your family, you will probably be the one person who holds your family unit and everyday activities together. You are the most important person in keeping all the other people in your life happy, healthy and safe – yet unless you start looking after yourself you are not going to keep every other aspect of your life ticking over. You need to raise yourself up the priority list, because unless you start looking after yourself, you are going to feel unhappy, less healthy and more run-down and you are not going to care for those important loved ones. This is one of the hardest things for many women to get their heads around: we need to embrace the fact that taking a little time out for ourselves – for exercise and healthy nutrition – will keep the whole thing moving. Once you understand this and put it into practice you will feel better and you will be able to ride the wave of stress much more successfully.

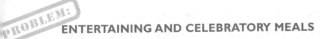

ENTERTAINING AND CELEBRATORY MEALS

Whether it is a classic Sunday roast, Christmas dinner, or a dinner party for friends, this type of meal is traditionally when we stock up and enjoy food and drink to excess. And to tell you the truth, this isn't a great problem. While a really excessive Christmas dinner with all the trimmings can add up to a total of nearly 7000 calories, it generally isn't that one day of excess that piles on the pounds, but rather the slow steady accumulation of calories over the whole holiday season, or the action you have taken over the course of the week. Remember, to gain a pound of weight you need to eat an additional 3500 calories a week – so that Christmas dinner should only be adding a couple of pounds. Think about it – if we want to lose a pound, we must try to achieve a calorie burn of 500 calories each day, therefore if we start eating an additional 500 calories a day, week in, week out, the pounds start to pile on and our health is negatively affected.

The physical activity habits that you learned in Habit Grooving start to become very important at these times. Remember, the weight that you will be in 24 months will not be determined by what you do for the next 24 hours or 24 days but by what you can keep doing for the next 24 months.

I started Joanna's plan a few months before Christmas, two years ago. I lost nearly a stone and I was really pleased. Over that first Christmas I was not very good with my habit grooving and gained back nine pounds. I was a bit disappointed. Over the next 12 months I continued to lose weight and decrease my body fat. I really got to grips with being consistent with my habits – especially increasing my physical activity levels. Yes, I had a few blips and I certainly was not good the whole time, so I approached the next Christmas with apprehension. When I weighed myself this time, I had only gained three pounds and I certainly ate all the Christmas goodies. Being consistent had worked – it was almost as if my body had got used to dealing with this extra load of calories and instead of saying 'I'll store this as fat', I was able to burn it off. **Judith, 53**

SOLUTION: **DAMAGE LIMITATION**

■ Operate a starch-free zone

See page 182 to find out how.

If you feel that you'll be selling your guests or family short by making healthier food choices, think again. Not only will you be doing everyone's health a favour, they won't even notice that you're implementing dietary strategies because the food you serve is so delicious! To prove the point, check out the Sunday lunch menu on page 233.

YOU CAN'T RESIST CHOCOLATE

WHY DO WE CRAVE CHOCOLATE?

There are times when nothing but chocolate will do. Chocolate cravings can occur because you are feeling lethargic and feel you need a sugar fix to give you an instant energy boost. Look to your lunch and your hydration levels. Check you are eating the right food ratios at lunchtime (see page 157) and increase your intake of slow-release carbohydrates. Cravings can also be psychological – you remember being given chocolate to soothe or reward you as a child and feel that it will make you feel better as an adult, too.

DAMAGE LIMITATION FOR CHOCOHOLICS

■ Phone a friend

Before you dive into that tempting family-sized bar of chocolate you bought for company, call a friend and tell her what you plan to do. It will help you weaken your 'need' to eat it.

■ Satisfy chocolate urges safely

When only chocolate will do, try these single servings, and don't keep them in the house:

Snack-size chocolate bar such as kiddies' chocolate animal bar

Finger of fudge

Low calorie hot chocolate drink

Chunks of frozen banana dipped in low-fat chocolate yoghurt

Thick and Creamy Chocolate Milk Shake

This recipe will help curb chocolate cravings – the milk provides essential calcium and the volume of the drink stretches your stomach, sending messages to the brain that you are full.

1 sachet low-fat chocolate instant drinking powder
Ice cubes
Half a banana, cut into chunks and frozen
280ml skimmed milk

Dissolve the chocolate sachet in a little hot water and fill up half the cup with cold water. Place in a blender, add some ice cubes, the frozen banana chunks and skimmed milk and blend for about 60 seconds. Pour into a glass and drink.

> Joanna's top tip: The frozen banana chunks are the vital ingredient here as they really thicken the shake and make you feel you are being very self-indulgent!

I found this recipe great – it really sorted out my chocolate cravings and I found it very filling and quick to make. I enjoyed it so much I used to have it every evening before I started cooking the family dinner – it really helped me to stop picking as I was preparing the meal.
Pam, 46, a self-confessed chocoholic, lost 14 pounds

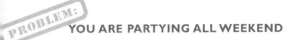

YOU ARE PARTYING ALL WEEKEND

Do you see Monday through until Friday lunchtime as your 'diet' days and the weekend as the chance to let your hair down, party and drink and eat what you want? If you are prepared to punish yourself all week to make up for the damage you do at the weekend, you are effectively living the No Air diet (see page vii) from Monday to Friday, week in, week out, and will probably be experiencing frustration at never really seeing the scales shift despite depriving yourself all week. If this sounds like you, and you feel that the only thing to do is stop partying altogether – well, you may be surprised, but I'm actually not going to tell you to do that. Firstly, you need to stop depriving yourself from Monday to Friday and start building in some little actions that mean you can party at the weekend. You'll need to ease back a bit but more importantly, you need to stop your erratic eating behaviour.

DAMAGE LIMITATION

■ The value of consistency

For you to see a change in the size of your body, you need to give each and every microscopic cell in your body a consistent message. Unless you are able to do this, you will not see much of a change in your body. Being consistent does not mean you have to be a goody two-shoes all the time – being consistent means that by grooving the habits you learned about in Section Two 80 per cent of the time, you will see a change in your body shape, you will have more energy and you can party at the weekends and not see the scales go sky high come Monday morning.

And the best thing is, the longer you are able to groove healthy habits, the more comfortable your body will become with occasional periods of excess. The abrupt increase in calories will not be laid down as fat and any weight gain will be more easily lost when you get back into your habit grooving – particularly if you take care to remain as active as possible.

I lost 28 pounds by following Joanna's plan and I kept it off – all my patients were amazed. Even when I went on holiday to Italy for a week and really partied and pigged out on the pasta, I only gained three pounds and a week after coming back off holiday I was back into my habit grooving and lost those three pounds – this really does work. **Tony, 46**

■ Don't rob Peter to pay Paul

If you know you are heading for a weekend of excess, don't starve yourself all week. Instead eat 300 calories less the day before your partying begins and be sure to fit in a structured exercise session. Then eat 300 calories less the day after your partying has finished. If your body feels up to it, do another structured exercise session but you may find it more appropriate to hit your step walking targets. Carry on being consistent through the rest of the week.

■ Double Starch Curfew

If you have a weekend of weddings, parties or other back-to-back social events operate a double Starch Curfew zone. Have a starch-free lunch and a Starch Curfew supper. I suggest this because the chances are your fat intake will be higher on these days, pushing up your calorie intake and it will be easier to minimize increased calorie intake by avoiding starch rather than trying to avoid the fatty foods.

■ Stay hydrated

After a weekend of excess you will feel tired – make sure you do not compound your feelings of tiredness by being dehydrated as well. Remember, drink little and often.

■ Veg up

Make yourself up a cauldron of vegetable soup to eat before you go out in the evening – this will curb your appetite and line your stomach.

Here's a great recipe for a hearty vegetable soup. If you don't want such a filling meal, look at the smoothie options on page 219.

Hearty Vegetable Soup

Serves 4

It's a good idea to make double and freeze for later.

2 teaspoons olive oil

1 onion, chopped

½ head cabbage, cut into 5cm pieces

2 carrots, cut into 2.5cm pieces

2 celery stalks, cut into 2.5cm pieces

1 courgette, cut into 2.5cm pieces

4 small red potatoes (with skin), cut into 2.5cm pieces

225g fresh mushrooms, sliced

6 tomatoes, peeled, seeded and diced

400ml chicken stock

15g fresh chopped basil

1 tbsp fresh thyme, chopped

½ teaspoon salt

¼ teaspoon freshly ground black pepper

Heat the oil in a large pan, over a medium heat. Add the onion and cabbage and sauté until tender, about 5 minutes. Add the carrots, celery, courgette, potatoes and mushrooms and simmer for 5 minutes.

Add the tomatoes, stock, basil, thyme, salt and pepper. Bring to the boil, reduce the heat to low and simmer until the potatoes are tender, about 30 minutes.

Note: If you are practising the Starch Curfew you can omit the potatoes.

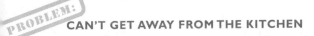

CAN'T GET AWAY FROM THE KITCHEN

If you spend a lot of your day in the kitchen then chances are you are faced with temptation continually. Maybe you clear the remains from your children's plates, nibble on snacks absentmindedly or just pick throughout the day instead of eating proper meals. Or perhaps you are so used to being in the kitchen you find yourself wandering in and out of the fridge with no specific reason at all. Contrary to popular belief, the calories you consume while standing next to the fridge *do* count!

I keep a bowl of fresh fruit salad in the fridge, also small fruit jellies for times when I fancy something sweet, or salad bits – cucumber, celery, radishes or the occasional pickled onion or walnut for a savoury snack. **Vanessa, 55**

DAMAGE LIMITATION

■ Plate patrol

If you can't resist hoovering the remains off everyone else's plate as you clear away then allocate someone to clear the table and clear the scraps straight into the rubbish bin. Then you can continue with your kitchen duties with temptation firmly out of the way.

■ Join in

If you really can't stop yourself from eating their leftovers, have a side salad for your starter and then put all the stored up leftovers on a plate and eat them properly as your main meal.

■ Role model

Think about it – you are your child's most influential role model. The visual and verbal images you give your children will have a direct impact on how they feel about food. So your actions are really important – making time to sit down with your children is not only important to help you keep your eating habits sensible and healthy but you are also giving them a fundamentally important message too.

■ Remind yourself

If you snack absentmindedly, wind a coloured plaster or wrap a piece of cotton around your 'eating hand' so every time you go to eat, you can see what you're doing. It will help you not to follow through on your impulse to eat, as well as provide insights into the types of 'triggers' that have you heading for the biscuit tin.

■ Think beyond baking biscuits

If you love your time in the kitchen and enjoy giving food as a gift, think beyond biscuits and cakes. Try infused vinegars and salsas. Avoid making baked foods that will be really hard to resist nibbling at, so if you volunteer to make something for a charity fete or school bizarre opt to make the seasoned oils and vinegars rather than the biscuits.

■ Never eat on two feet

Resolve never to eat on two feet. If you can't stop nibbling – that's fine, but make sure whatever it is you are going to sample, you sit down to eat and don't wander around. Make this your mantra and you could be surprised at how many calories you save.

■ Kitchen sleep-walking

If you find yourself walking into the kitchen when you really have no need to and raiding the fridge, why not shut that kitchen door once you have completed everything you need to do in there and put a large piece of tape over the door. That way, when you have to go into the kitchen you can make sure you are giving in because you need to rather than just for the sake of it.

PROBLEM:

WEEKENDS LET YOU DOWN

You find it easy to be 'good all week' but at the weekend, when there's less of a routine, you let it all go.

SOLUTION:

DAMAGE LIMITATION

■ Try the two-meal tool

At weekends, we often have two meals quite close together.

Many of us have breakfast late and then lunch an hour or two later. Both these meals will also tend to be a bit bigger than you would have during the week. Save calories by having just two meals a day at weekends, breakfast and dinner, and opt for a snack in between. See *In Your Mouth in 5 Mins* (page 224) for substantial snacks that are healthy and nutritious.

■ Cook on a full stomach

If you have to bake or prepare for a dinner party, try to do it when you are full, after a meal or in the morning. Your willpower will be higher and you will be less prone to nibble the whole time.

■ Stretch your lunch

If you know you always get hungry in the afternoon, split your lunch into two sittings. Eat half at your normal lunchtime and the remaining half in the afternoon – but make sure you sit down for it rather than eating it at the fridge.

PROBLEM: TIME OF THE MONTH

Many women find that try as they might, they just can't resist those food cravings at the time of the month. Studies show that in the two weeks leading up to your period, your metabolic rate actually increases by about 140 calories. So now you know why you are more hungry and want to eat more food. The problem is that chocolate bar you are craving will, on average, provide 250 calories, so that means an excess of 110 calories already!

SOLUTION:

DAMAGE LIMITATION

■ Opt for 100-calorie snacks
■ 2 squares Dairy Milk chocolate
■ 2 oatcakes
■ any piece of fruit
■ 20 almonds
■ 8 dried apricots
■ 1 small pot low-fat yoghurt and a small banana
■ a palmful of sunflower and pumpkin seeds
■ 2 rice cakes topped with cottage cheese
■ half a small avocado filled with salsa

■ Allocate a binge zone

If you really feel you are not going to be able to resist a binge, then define your zone. Allocate yourself a time when you can binge, for example 9–11 p.m., but during that time eat your fill of the lowest-calorie foods possible – try bowls of water-packed fruits like strawberries or melon, or some steamed veg. You will be full, but will have more chance to stay within your calorie limit.

■ Take time out

When you feel your eating is out of control, you need to

disconnect temporarily from the activity of eating so you can decide whether you want to continue. Remember you are in control, but you need to give yourself some space to realize this. Get up from the table, brush your teeth, or stop and clean a room in the house. Do what ever it takes to give yourself a break. Your brain needs time to register it is full and studies have shown this takes about 20 minutes from the act of eating to your brain registering it is full.

■ Switch the taste sensation

You can help stop a binge in its tracks by switching to a completely different food the moment you catch yourself at the point of bingeing. So if you have started to polish off a carton of ice cream, put the carton away and pull out a bag of fruit or carrot sticks. It will give you an opportunity to create some distance from the easy-eating, high-calorie food.

PROBLEM:

TRAVELLING

Travelling and being away from your normal environment can be a killer: dealing with different time zones, different food choices, perhaps deciphering different food cultures and languages and, of course, being just plain tired. Of course, you don't have to travel abroad to confront the perils of taking time out – just about any kind of trip can interfere with our good intentions.

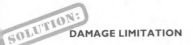

DAMAGE LIMITATION

■ Pre-order your meal

If flying, pre-order a special meal. This is quite easy to do and the airlines are quite happy to do this when asked, except they tend not to make it public knowledge. There is a wide range of special meals you can order – low fat, low calorie, low cholesterol, kosher, vegetarian, to name a few. From my personal experience, different airlines use different criteria to define these different meals. I have found, however, that the veggie option is almost invariably higher in fat than other choices as it is usually based on cheese! So don't pre-order this. So far I have not come across an airline that will specifically pre-pare you a Starch Curfew dinner – but keep asking, one day they will say yes! Failing that, I'd recommend you request a low calorie meal. I suggest this rather than the low-fat meal as I have found this often turns out to be a low cholesterol meal that still has an overall high fat content. The low-calorie options I have had tend to be a better meal all round. And remember to say no to the bread roll and drink plenty of water.

■ Prior protein

Prior to starting out, make sure your last meal has a good balance of protein and starch, so you feel satisfied and motivated as opposed to lethargic. Even athletes travelling around the world to compete use this strategy to minimize the detrimental effects of travelling on their performance.

This pre-flight strategy is also very useful if you are embarking on a long car journey. In this case, you may prefer to just have a smaller protein meal with lots of vegetables and fruit. Remember not to eat too much or your blood sugar levels will rise too quickly and you'll end up feeling lethargic.

■ Blinker out the cash point

Resolve not to loiter by the sweets at the garage counter. If you must buy something, grab some chewing chum and a bottle of water or hard-boiled sweets that take longer to eat, rather than a bag of jelly beans or chocolates.

I found I had really got into the habit of not just paying for the petrol but also for a car supply of journey snacks – I used the children as an excuse, and then I found it was me that was devouring them and not the kids! So now I resolve only to buy myself some gum and save the sweets for the kids. As soon as I get in the car I start chewing it so I can't be tempted by the kids' jelly babies!
Lucinda, 37

■ Pack your pedometer

You may not feel like exercising as soon as you arrive at your destination but do try to move your body – resolve to get 4000 steps on that pedometer as soon as possible. It's a great way to explore your destination, and it'll help you get rid of that 'travelling fatigue' feeling. If you are on a business trip and your structured exercise sessions are just not going to happen, resolve to get in your daily 10,000 steps – even if it means getting up a little earlier to get them done.

■ Avoid excess snack baggage

If you are at a bar, or are offered nibbles with your pre-flight dinner, say NO – they are laden with salt and calories and will only add to your excess baggage rather than helping you to go first class with your health!

■ Operate the Starch Curfew wherever possible

It works at home and it works just as well when you're away. Take the opportunity to try varieties of fruit and vegetables that aren't available at home and restrict starchy foods to lunchtimes.

I travel nearly 200 days of the year. I entertain clients for lunch in one country and in another for dinner – my life sounds glamorous but with the weight I was gaining, my appearance certainly wasn't! I had no energy for exercise and the weight was piling on. Once I started operating the Starch Curfew I lost a lot of weight. I found I had more energy and I did not have to feel awkward when ordering in front of clients at a restaurant over a business dinner. No one ever knew I was on a 'diet'. To me it is not a diet, it is a strategy and, as a businessman, I can really get my head around that. The Starch Curfew works! **Richard, 48**

GET A GRIP, HABIT GROOVING OR DAMAGE LIMITATION?

When you picked up this book, you were probably feeling motivated and ready to put your weight loss plan into action. However, over the weeks of your programme there may have been times when your motivation waned a little or life got very hectic and you weren't able to put into practice as many of the habit-grooving action points as you would have liked. Well, that's life. It's meant to be enjoyed, so let's embrace the things we can do and not beat ourselves up for the things we can't. Every small thing you do matters, so be proud of your efforts. Now that you've read through all the sections of the book, you have probably realized that at some times more than others, you will face challenges and difficulties in maintaining your new healthy habits. It is important to plan ahead and identify when you may experience these difficulties and approach them with the right attitude.

To help you do this, I suggest you identify your weeks by the following categories:

PROGRESSIVE

A progressive week is a week when you feel motivated, you are clear about what you need to do and you are able to put all your tasks in action. You feel confident about being able to fit in your exercise and follow the nutritional guidelines.

HABIT GROOVING

This is when you know it will be a little challenging to get all the tasks completed. Maybe the challenges are due to a deadline you know you have to complete at work and you have to work late, or a member of your family or a friend is unwell and you have to look after them. These are weeks when you may not be able to complete all your tasks, but you can still consolidate your efforts and think about grooving your healthy lifestyle habits. For example, focus on always drinking your water each day and completing your walks. You are still making progress in these weeks, as habit grooving is a crucial process not just in realizing your weight loss goals, but also in keeping the weight off.

DAMAGE LIMITATION

This is when life gets really manic. Maybe you are moving house, changing jobs, going to lots of parties, or the washing machine floods your home ... All of these situations can really throw you off your good intentions. It is quite common for these situations to make you feel like giving up for that week and starting a week later. You may be thinking – I'll forget about this week and start again in earnest next week when things are quieter. This is not a good idea, as next week will come and you will feel as if you have to undo the damage you have done from the previous week. The secret of damage limitation is acknowledging things may be difficult in the week ahead but planning a few habit grooving action points that will help you work towards your goals. These need to be small, achievable things. For example, you don't have time to fit in your walk, but you decide to get up for 60 seconds every hour and do some exercises. You know you won't have time to cook so you check out the diet plan and stock up on some ready-prepared stand-bys such as packet sushi, chiller-cabinet soups or prepared fruit salads. This way you will still be feeling positive about your actions and when things calm down, you won't feel as if you have to start again to continue working towards your goals.

As you continue with this programme it is a good idea to look ahead and identify whether the coming week will be a Progressive, Habit Grooving or Damage Limitation one. We are not always in the ideal situation of being able to do everything right, but the good news is, we don't have to do everything right all the time in order to get – and stay – fit and healthy. So be realistic about what you can achieve, continue to use and groove the skills you've learned in this programme and you will not just lose the weight, but keep it off.

RECIPES AND RESOURCES

In this section you will find lots of ideas to expand your repertoire of healthy recipes. You can, of course, continue to use the recipes featured in the 14-day *Get a Grip* plan – the recipes featured here are not designed to replace these, simply to give you more choice once you have completed the initial diet and are ready to take up healthy eating permanently. To encourage you to keep up your intake of liquid-based foods I have included a number of ideas for soups and smoothies. You will also find quick and easy snacks and Starch Curfew meals, as well as some recipes for entertaining – including a Sunday lunch menu and some dips and canapés for parties.

SOUPS

Soups are filling and healthy and should definitely be added to the list when you're thinking about what to have for lunch. There's no need to spend ages chopping up veg though. Many of the following soup recipes use quick, convenient ingredients without compromising taste – for instance ready-made chilled soups as a base and packs of ready-prepared veg to give added flavour and nutritional value. For a Starch Curfew meal, check that any soup you use as a base doesn't include potatoes, wheat flour or pasta.

Spicy Corn and Fish Chowder

Serves 2–3

1 carton spicy corn chowder
1 piece (about 300g) smoked haddock –
    use a piece of unsmoked fish if
    preferred
280ml skimmed milk
half a head of broccoli, cut into bite-size
    florets or ¼ cauliflower cut into florets

Info per serving:
Calories: 242.0
Fat: 5.8g
Saturated Fat: 2.5g
Protein: 21.5g
Carbohydrate: 24.4g

Preheat the oven 200°C/400°F/Gas mark 6.

Put the fish in shallow ovenproof dish and pour the

milk over the fish. Cook in the oven for 10 minutes. Remove from the dish and break the flesh up into bite-size chunks (checking to see there are no bones at the same time).

Microwave the broccoli or cauliflower in a little water for 3 minutes on high. Pour the soup into a pan and heat through. At the last minute, add the smoked haddock and vegetables and stir in well.

Wild Mushroom Soup

Serves 2–3

1 carton wild mushroom soup
light olive oil
3–4 dark-gilled mushrooms, thinly sliced
1 teaspoon freeze-dried parsley or thyme
good handful of bean sprouts

> **Info per serving:**
> Calories: 133.0
> Fat: 6.8g
> Saturated Fat: 3.3g
> Protein: 6.6g
> Carbohydrate: 11.2g

Gently heat the soup in a saucepan.

Meanwhile, stir-fry the mushroom in ½ teaspoon of oil on a high heat for 1 minute. Add the herbs and bean sprouts and cook for 30–40 seconds. Divide the heated soup between the bowls and pile the mushrooms and bean sprouts in the centre.

Carrot and Coriander Soup

Serves 2–3

1 carton carrot and coriander soup
(Covent Garden is best)
200ml skimmed milk
1 tablespoon low-fat Greek or natural
yoghurt
fresh coriander
freshly ground black pepper

Info per serving:
Calories: 91.0
Fat: 2.70g
Saturated Fat: trace
Protein: 6.0g
Carbohydrate: 10.6g

Empty the soup into a large bowl. Add the milk and chill. Divide the soup between the serving bowls, put a small dollop of yoghurt in the centre and sprinkle over some fresh coriander and pepper.

Very Quick Cucumber and Mint Soup

Serves 4

1 cucumber
250g low fat Greek-style yoghurt
4 tablespoons skimmed milk
2 garlic cloves, crushed
2 tablespoons chopped fresh mint
2 tablespoons white wine vinegar
salt and freshly ground black pepper
some sprigs of mint for decoration

Info per serving:
Calories: 85.2
Fat: 4.0g
Saturated Fat: 0.1g
Protein: 6.0g
Carbohydrate: 6.7g

Cut the ends off the cucumber and chop roughly. Place in a blender or food processor with the rest of the ingredients and whizz until smooth. Check the seasoning and chill until needed. Serve with a sprig of mint floating on top.

Spicy Carrot Soup with a Floating Salad

Serves 4

1 large onion, finely chopped

2 teaspoons minced garlic (available in a
   tube or jar)

2 teaspoons minced ginger (available in a
   tube or jar)

1 tablespoon medium curry paste

420g can yellow split peas, drained and rinsed

450g carrots, coarsely grated

1.2 litres vegetable stock

1 tablespoon groundnut oil

2 teaspoons onion seeds

1 teaspoon curry paste

300g bag stir-fry vegetables (most supermarkets stock them)

> **Info per serving:**
> Calories: 332.0
> Fat: 2.8g
> Saturated Fat: 0.9g
> Protein: 19.9g
> Carbohydrate: 51.9g

Dry-fry the onion and half the garlic and ginger in a large non-stick pan for 2 minutes – if it catches add a drop or two of water. Stir in the tablespoon of curry paste and cook for a further minute. Stir in the split peas, carrots and stock. Bring to the boil and simmer for 25 minutes. Transfer it all to a blender or food processor and blitz until smooth. Season well.

Heat the oil in a wok or frying pan and fry the onion seeds until they start to pop. Add the remaining garlic and ginger, the 1 teaspoon of curry paste and the pack of vegetables. Stir-fry for 2 minutes. Add salt to taste.

Divide the soup between the serving bowls and pile a little of the salad in the middle of each.

Tom Yum Soup with Mushrooms

Serves 4

This takes a little preparation but it's worth it for a really tasty, very low-cal soup.

2 stalks lemon grass (peel them down to
    the tender whitish centres)
1.2 litres vegetable stock
5cm piece fresh root ginger, grated
1 fresh red chilli, seeded and finely sliced
    (wear rubber gloves or wash your
    hands well afterwards)
¼ teaspoon freshly ground black pepper
2 tablespoons soy sauce
juice of 1 lime
8 button mushrooms, quartered
2 spring onions, shredded
small handful of fresh coriander leaves

Info per serving:
Calories: 48.0
Fat: 0.6g
Saturated Fat: 0.2g
Protein: 3.5g
Carbohydrate: 8.5g

Bash the lemon grass stalks with a rolling pin to crush them and then cut into 2.5cm pieces. Put the vegetable stock into a pan and bring it to the boil. Add the crushed lemon grass, cover and simmer on a low heat for 10 minutes. Remove the lemon grass with a slotted spoon and discard.

Add the ginger, chilli, black pepper, soy sauce and lime juice to the stock. Simmer for a further 3 minutes then add the mushrooms. Remove from the heat, cover and leave for 10 minutes. Serve with spring onions and coriander.

Parsnip Soup with Spinach

Serves 4

1 teaspoon olive oil
1 onion, sliced
1 teaspoon ground coriander
900g parsnips, peeled and coarsely
   chopped
1.2 litres vegetable stock
salt and freshly ground black pepper

> **Info per serving:**
> Calories: 290.0
> Fat: 8.0g
> Saturated Fat: 1.2g
> Protein: 5.4g
> Carbohydrate: 48.0g

For the spinach:
1 teaspoon olive oil
2 garlic cloves, sliced
225g washed baby spinach

Heat the oil in a large pan and fry the onions and coriander for 3 minutes until soft and translucent. Add the prepared parsnips and fry gently for 4 minutes.

Pour in the vegetable stock, season and bring to the boil. Cover and simmer on a low heat for about 30 minutes until the parsnips are tender. Cool for a few minutes and transfer to a blender or food processor and whizz until smooth. (You may need to do this in batches). Return the soup to the pan and reheat gently.

Meanwhile, in a frying pan, fry the garlic for a minute and then add the spinach until it just starts to wilt. Spoon the soup into bowls and top with the garlicky spinach.

Quick Curried Sweetcorn Soup

Serves 2

1 teaspoon olive oil
1 small onion, chopped
2 garlic cloves, crushed
1 teaspoon curry powder
225g frozen sweetcorn
150ml dry white wine
450ml vegetable stock
2 tablespoons half fat crème fraiche
salt and freshly ground black pepper

Info per serving:
Calories: 265.0
Fat: 10.4g
Saturated Fat: 2.7g
Protein: 5.8g
Carbohydrate: 33.5g

Heat the oil in a large pan and cook the onion, garlic and curry powder over a low heat for 5 minutes.

Add all the remaining ingredients except the crème fraiche. Bring to the boil and simmer for 10 minutes.

Stir in the crème fraiche and transfer to a blender or food processor and whizz until smooth. Taste and adjust seasoning.

Very Easy Pea and Watercress Soup

Serves 4

1 tablespoon olive oil
1 large onion, chopped
500ml vegetable stock
350g frozen peas
75g bag watercress

Info per serving:
Calories: 116.0
Fat: 3.9g
Saturated Fat: 0.6g
Protein: 5.8g
Carbohydrate: 15.4g

Heat the oil in the pan, add the onion and cook until soft – 3–4 minutes. Pour in the stock and bring to the boil, then lower the heat, add the frozen peas and simmer for 3 minutes.

Pick out and discard the thicker stems of watercress and stir the rest into the soup. Cook for about a minute, transfer to a blender or food processor and whizz until almost smooth – there should be a little texture.

SMOOTHIES

Smoothies are great to experiment at home with – when you have complete control over what goes into them. All you need is a blender and you're away. Suck and see is the motto – try loads of different combinations and see what you like. If you or your children have trouble eating enough fruit, smoothies are the perfect answer.

Buy fruit in your local markets, particularly in the summer months when there is so much choice and the prices are lower than the supermarkets.

Smoothies are great at lunchtime or have them mid-morning or mid-afternoon. For optimum flavour and nutritional value, smoothies are best drunk immediately after making them.

Mango and Peach Smoothie

Makes 2 glasses

1 mango, peeled and flesh coarsely
   chopped
3 peaches, pitted and coarsely chopped
3 tablespoons low-fat yoghurt

Info per serving:
Calories: 185.0
Fat: 0.9g
Saturated Fat: 0.4g
Protein: 3.5g
Carbohydrate: 45.5g

Blend until smooth.

Orange, Pineapple and Raspberry Fizz

Makes 4 glasses

juice of 3–4 oranges
½ a large pineapple, peeled and coarsely
    chopped
1 punnet of raspberries
250ml sparkling mineral water

Info per serving:
Calories: 148.0
Fat: 1.0g
Saturated Fat: trace
Protein: 10.0g
Carbohydrate: 22.0g

Blend the fruit until smooth. Strain through a fine plastic sieve and add the sparkling water, stirring in gently.

Apricot, Banana and Honeydew Melon Nectar

Makes 2–3 glasses

5 ripe apricots, pitted and coarsely
    chopped
1 banana, peeled and broken up into
    chunks
half a medium-sized honeydew melon,
    seeded and cut into chunks

Info per serving:
Calories: 164.0
Fat: 1.0g
Saturated Fat: trace
Protein: 10.0g
Carbohydrate: 26.0g

Place the fruit in a blender and blend until smooth.

Banana, Kiwi and Orange Nectar

Makes 2 glasses

1 banana, peeled and broken into chunks
1 kiwi, peeled and halved
juice of 3 oranges

Info per serving:
Calories: 141.0
Fat: 0.8g
Saturated Fat: 0.1g
Protein: 2.3g
Carbohydrate: 33.4g

Place the fruit and juice in a blender and blend until smooth.

"IN YOUR MOUTH IN 5 MINS" SNACKS

These are substantial snacks that can also double as light lunches. When hunger attacks, chocolate bars, biscuits or just good old toast and butter can seem so much quicker than preparing something nutritious, so these snacks have been designed with speed in mind. All are low calorie and designed to curb your hunger, stimulate your concentration and boost your blood sugar levels.

It's as easy as pie, all you need to do is choose one item from the 'bases' column and one from the 'toppings' column. Put them together and away you go!

Bases

2 Ryvita crispbreads

1 slice malted wheat bread

1 slice granary bread

1 slice German rye bread

1 slice sourdough bread

1 medium wholemeal pitta bread

1 slice mixed seed bread

Toppings

1. 30g smoked salmon, 10g light cream cheese, ½ chopped spring onion plus pickled dill cucumbers

2. 100g skinned chicken breasts, 1 teaspoon pesto, 3 shredded lettuce leaves, 1 sliced tomato plus seasoning

3. 125g cottage cheese, ½ chopped spring onion, 2 slices black forest ham (all fat removed) plus seasoning

4. 50g quark, 1 heaped teaspoon creamed horseradish, 100g cooked beef slices plus 1 teaspoon American sweet onion mustard (Sainsbury's)

5. 50g quark, 1 teaspoon horseradish, 75g skinned smoked mackerel, 2 shredded lettuce leaves plus chives

6. 125g drained tuna in brine, ½ chopped spring onion, 1 chopped celery stick plus 1 teaspoon low-cal mayo

7. 1 sliced cooked beetroot, 100g low-fat tzatziki (yoghurt with cucumber) plus ½ chopped spring onion

8. 100g reduced-fat houmous, 1 grated carrot plus ½ chopped spring onion

9. 100g cooked and peeled prawns, 2 tablespoons natural yoghurt, 1 tablespoon mango chutney, ½ teaspoon curry paste, plus 2 shredded lettuce leaves

10. 100g drained tuna in brine, 150g cooked chickpeas, ⅓ chopped red onion plus 1 teaspoon low-cal mayo

11. 100g packet chicken tikka cubes, 100g low-fat tzatziki, plus 2 shredded lettuce leaves

EMERGENCY RATION PACK

Keeping a stock of ready-prepared emergency fruit and veg rations in a plastic box in the fridge is a great way for avoiding the temptation of unhealthy snacking. They're also good served with lunch.

Try these:

- peeled and quartered carrots
- sticks of celery
- sticks of cucumber
- washed radishes
- punnets of soft fruits and packs of prepared pineapple and melon

You can eat them on their own or team with a healthy dip. Bought dips are great but it's much cheaper and quick to make some yourself. Check out the dip recipes on page 248 for some inspiration.

"ON YOUR PLATE IN 15 MINS" STARCH CURFEW DINNERS

You walk in the door from work, you're tired, hungry and you need to eat. Well, here's the answer – six Starch Curfew dinners that can be on your table in less than 15 minutes. Remember to serve your Starch Curfew dinners with unlimited vegetables from the list on page 48.

Quick Glazed Pork Loin Chops

Serves 4

2 tablespoons orange smooth marmalade
1 tablespoon Dijon mustard
½ teaspoon Chinese five spice powder
4 pork chops

Info per serving:
Calories: 294.0
Fat: 13.0g
Saturated Fat: 5.0g
Protein: 35.3g
Carbohydrate: 6.9g

Preheat the grill to medium. Mix together the marmalade, mustard and five spice powder. Put the chops on a grill pan and brush the glaze over them. Cook through until meat is no longer pink, about 12–15 minutes, turning over halfway through cooking. Baste with more glaze if needed. This dish is also suitable for barbecuing.

Quick Thai Chicken and Coconut Curry

Serves 4

1–2 tablespoons red or green Thai curry
    paste (now widely available in jars)
450g chicken breasts, cubed
salt and freshly ground black pepper
225g broccoli, broken up into florets
200ml carton reduced-fat coconut cream
good handful fresh coriander, roughly chopped

Info per serving:
Calories: 311.8
Fat: 13.9g
Saturated Fat: 9.0g
Protein: 38.4g
Carbohydrate: 8.5g

Mix the curry paste in a saucepan with 2 tablespoons of water. Add the cubed chicken, seasoning and 150ml of water. Bring to the boil, lower the heat and simmer for 12–15 minutes until chicken is tender.

Meanwhile, cook the broccoli in some boiling salted water, drain and add to the chicken along with the coconut cream. Simmer gently for 2–3 minutes. Sprinkle over the coriander.

Other vegetables can be added, such as sugar snap peas, courgettes or green beans.

Microwave Cod and Cabbage

Serves 4

1 tsp light olive oil
2 slices unsmoked lean back bacon,
   chopped
1 small Savoy cabbage, shredded
150ml vegetable stock
4 cod fillets, skinned
salt and freshly ground black pepper

> **Info per serving:**
> Calories: 155.6
> Fat: 3.7g
> Saturated Fat: 1.0g
> Protein: 27.5g
> Carbohydrate: 1.6g

Heat the oil in a non-stick frying pan and when it starts to smoke add the bacon, tossing for 3–5 minutes until crisp.

Stir in the cabbage, pour over the stock and cook for a further 3 minutes, stirring all the time until almost tender. Transfer to a microwaveable dish.

Lay the fish on top of the cabbage, and season. Cover with clingfilm and cook on high in a microwave for 5 minutes until the fish is cooked (the flesh starts to turn opaque).

Cheater's Beef Bourguignon with Chickpeas

Serves 2

1 pack Waitrose Bistro range Beef Bourguignon
1 pack Waitrose Bistro Green Vegetable Trio
400g can chickpeas
150g carton half-fat crème fraiche
1 garlic clove, crushed
salt and freshly ground black pepper

Cook the beef and the vegetables according to the instructions on the packs.

Pour the chickpeas with half the juice from the can into a food processor. Add 1 tablespoon crème fraiche and the crushed garlic and season well. Blitz until smooth. Heat the puree in a pan and serve on each plate with the vegetables and the beef stacked on top.

Quick Lamb and Spring Onion Stir-Fry

Serves 4

4 tablespoons soy sauce

4 tablespoons sherry

1 tablespoon sesame oil

2 teaspoons wine vinegar

1 tablespoon groundnut oil

2 garlic cloves, thinly sliced

bunch of spring onions, sliced into 5cm diagonal lengths

450g lamb fillet, sliced thinly across the grain

> **Info per serving:**
> Calories: 255.0
> Fat: 12.6g
> Saturated Fat: 3.1g
> Protein: 25.8g
> Carbohydrate: 5.3g

Mix together the soy sauce, sherry, sesame oil, vinegar and 4 tablespoons of water. On a high flame, heat a wok or frying pan with the oil and add the garlic. After a few seconds, add the lamb and stir-fry for 1–2 minutes until browned. Stir in the soy mixture and allow to bubble briefly. Add the spring onions and cook for a few more seconds until they just begin to soften. Serve with some steamed broccoli.

Quick Cod and Tomato Stew

Serves 4

2 chopped onions
1 tsp light olive oil
400g can chopped tomatoes
1 tablespoon soy sauce
1 teaspoon fresh or ½ teaspoon freeze-
   dried thyme
salt and freshly-ground black pepper
skinless cod fillets

Info per serving:
Calories: 185.8
Fat: 2.1g
Saturated Fat: 0.3g
Protein: 20.7g
Carbohydrate: 23.6g

Fry the onions in light olive oil until soft and just turning brown.

Stir in the tomatoes, soy sauce, thyme and seasoning. Bring to the boil, stir well and simmer uncovered until sauce reduces and slightly thickens.

Slide the fish into the pan, cover with a lid and cook gently until the fish is tender, about 5 minutes. Serve with lots of shredded steamed cabbage.

SUMMER SUNDAY ENTERTAINING MENU

It's a beautiful Summer's day and you plan to have friends round for dinner at the weekend. Here's a great menu plan that's nutritious, healthy and follows Starch Curfew.

Serves 4

Beginning with...
Artichokes Vinaigrette

Followed by...
Lemon, Thyme and Garlic Stuffed Roast Chicken with Roasted Vegetables and Wok-fried Greens

And finishing with...
Apple and Blackberry 'without the pie' with Greek Yoghurt Chantilly

INGREDIENTS FOR THE WHOLE MENU

- **4 globe artichokes** – should be a nice olive green colour with no black spots. They are a bit fiddly but well worth it if you like your veg!
- **Vinaigrette** – can be bought ready made or make your own using Dijon mustard, white wine vinegar, olive oil and a crushed garlic clove.

1.5kg free-range chicken – you don't need to bother with an over-priced organic bird but free rangers are worth the extra expense.

Bunch of thyme and a bulb of garlic – strip the leaves off half of the thyme sprigs and peel about 10 cloves of garlic but leave them whole.

Half an onion, peeled

1 lemon, cut in half

4 courgettes, halved lengthways and then halved again if thick

1 large aubergine, cut into big chunks

3 red peppers, seeded and cut into chunks

3 red onions, halved and quartered

1 packet fresh asparagus (if in season), cut in half diagonally

1 fennel bulb, trimmed of outer leaves and cut into quarters

2 packs spring onions, trimmed but kept whole

light olive oil

1 pack greens, trimmed, washed and shredded

dash of Japanese soy sauce

4 Bramley apples, washed and cored

runny honey

Demerara sugar

punnet of blackberries, washed

pot of Greek yoghurt, flavoured with a little caster sugar and vanilla extract

Artichokes Vinaigrette

This can be cooked and chilled the day before.

With each artichoke, first cut the stalk off as close to the leaves as possible. Using a pair of scissors, snip the pointed bit off each leaf, working from top to bottom. Pull off the reedy-looking leaves from the base and then give the artichokes a good rinse in cold water. Cook in lots of boiling salted water (to prevent discolouration don't use an iron or aluminium pan) with a little drop of vinegar. Cook them with the lid on, on a medium heat, for about 30–50 minutes, depending on the size. They are cooked when the leaves come out when tugged gently. Put them in a colander upside down to drain them well and cover and chill when cool.

To serve, place each cooled artichoke on a big plate and season with flaky salt and pepper. Drizzle vinaigrette over each one and have some in a pot if extra is needed. To eat them, pull off the leaves individually and, with your teeth, scrape off the creamy flesh from the bottom of each leaf. When the leaves become thin, diaphanous and reedy, pull them all off and discard. Gently, with a knife, scrape off and discard the hairy choke protecting the heart. Keep a bowl of warm water with a lemon slice to wash your fingers at the table.

Lemon, Thyme and Garlic Roast Chicken

Preheat oven to 180°C/350°F/Gas mark 5.

First pull out any unwanted bits of fat clinging to the inside of the chicken.

Loosen the skin covering the breast meat carefully with your fingers, trying hard not to pierce the skin.

Crush 5 cloves of garlic and mix them in a bowl with a handful of thyme leaves and 2 teaspoons of salt. Gently push the garlic herb paste in between the flesh and the skin as far and as evenly as possible. Put the remaining whole garlic cloves inside the cavity of the bird along with the thyme sprigs, half a lemon and the half onion. Place the bird in a roasting tin, squeeze over the juice from the remaining lemon half and season well, inside and out, with sea salt and ground black pepper.

Put the chicken in the oven on the middle shelf and roast for about 1 hour, until the juices run clear when the flesh is pierced. Remove the chicken to a serving plate, pour off the fat from the roasting tin and discard. Loosen the juices with a little water or stock if preferred over a low flame for a couple of minutes.

Roasted Vegetables

About 15 minutes after the chicken goes in the oven, the vegetables can go in, on the top shelf. Place the prepared vegetables, except the asparagus (they take less time to cook) in a roasting tray, making sure the onion in particular is evenly distributed in the tin. Drizzle some olive oil over in a thin trickle. Season well and make sure they are all well coated. Check them every 15 minutes, turning them and giving the tin a good shake to loosen any vegetables sticking to the bottom. They will be ready when they turn a light caramel colour and are cooked through – about 45 minutes, depending on the intensity of the oven. The asparagus can either be added to the rest of the vegetables with 20 minutes to go, or can be cooked separately using the same method.

If you want to use root vegetables instead, carrots, onions, leeks and parsnips are a good combination – cooked using exactly the same method and, as long as they are all cut into roughly the same size chunks, taking about the same amount of time.

Wok-fried Greens

Heat a wok until smoking and add 1 teaspoon of olive oil, swilling it around. Add the shredded greens and keep them moving around the wok by stirring all the time. Add about a tablespoon of soy sauce, coating the leaves as much as possible. When the greens have just a little bite to them and have reduced and wilted down a bit, they are ready to serve.

Serve some greens piled into the centre of the plate. On top, lay some roasted vegetables, making sure everybody gets a good even mix. Lay the chicken on top and drizzle some of the pan juices over the top.

Apple and Blackberry 'without the pie' with Greek Yoghurt Chantilly

Preheat the oven to 180°C/350°F/Gas mark 5.

Place the cored apples into a small roasting tin. Add 2 tablespoons water to the base of the tin. Put some Demerara sugar into a bowl and roll the still wet blackberries into the sugar to get a good coating. Push as many sugared blackberries as possible down into the centre of each apple. When all four apples are prepared, drizzle some runny honey over each and put them on the middle shelf, once the chicken has come out. Roast the apples for 30–40 minutes, depending on their size.

Serve warm or cold with a good dollop of the sweetened and flavoured Greek yoghurt on the side.

FISH OPTION MAIN COURSE

Italian Cod (or monkfish) with Garlic Tomatoes

Serves 4

2 unpeeled garlic cloves

1 tablespoon olive oil

100g black olives

900g tomatoes, preferably plum – keep
   them whole with stalks

2 red chillies, seeded and roughly chopped

3 tablespoons fresh pesto

2 boneless, skinless cod fillets or monkfish tails, approximately
   450g each in weight

grated rind of 1 lemon

12 slices of prosciutto or Serrano ham – fat removed

Info per serving:
Calories: 392.0
Fat: 12.0g
Saturated Fat: 3.6g
Protein: 50.0g
Carbohydrate: 14.9g

Preheat the oven to 200°C/400°F/Gas mark 6.

Put 2 tablespoons of oil in a roasting tin with the garlic and roast for 15 minutes. Add the tomatoes, olives and chillies to the tin, mixing them in with the oil and add seasoning.

Spread the pesto over one side of a cod fillet and sprinkle on some lemon juice and seasoning. Lay the other cod fillet on top and loosely wrap the ham slices around the fish, tucking in the edges on either side. Lightly drizzle with olive oil and put the cod on a grill rack over the tin. Roast the fish for 20 minutes, when the fish should be cooked and the tomatoes starting to break up.

Transfer the fish to a serving plate. Mash the two garlic cloves into the pan juices and throw away the tough outer skins. Serve the fish with the pan juices drizzled over the top. Serve with sautéed courgettes and a green salad.

VEGETARIAN OPTION MAIN COURSE

Baked Aubergine and Fennel with Shallots

This recipe is suitable for vegans if the Parmesan is omitted.

Serves 6

2 large garlic cloves, crushed

2 tablespoons sun-dried tomato paste

6 tablespoons olive oil

1 tablespoon balsamic vinegar

1 tablespoon lemon juice

3 fennel bulbs

1 large aubergine

12 shallots

400g can chickpeas, drained

75g freshly grated Parmesan

1 bunch spring onions, sliced diagonally in 5mm slices

Coarsely ground black pepper

Info per serving:
Calories: 325.2
Fat: 19.4g
Saturated Fat: 4.3g
Protein: 11.1g
Carbohydrate: 29.0g

Preheat oven to 200°C/400°F/Gas mark 6.

Into a screwtop jar put the crushed garlic, tomato paste, 2 tablespoons olive oil, the vinegar, lemon juice and black pepper. Give it a good shake.

Top and tail the fennel. Keep back the feathery leaves for later and discard any blemished outer leaves. Slice thinly lengthways and put into a bowl. Top and tail the aubergine. Halve lengthways and cut into chunks. Peel and quarter the shallots and add to the fennel and aubergine, along with the chickpeas. Add the garlic mixture and mix into the vegetables thoroughly.

Put the vegetables into a roasting tin and cook for 30 minutes. Sprinkle with the Parmesan and cook for a further 10 minutes until melted and golden.

Roughly chop the reserved feathery fennel and scatter over the vegetables. Drizzle over the remaining olive oil before serving.

CANAPÉS AND HEALTHY PARTY DIPS

Smoked Salmon Rounds

Makes around 18

6 slices pumpernickel or German rye
   bread
300g pack low-fat cream cheese
chives, snipped into 5mm using scissors
300g smoked salmon
red spring onions, sliced very thinly

Info per serving:
Calories: 65.9
Fat: 1.8g
Saturated Fat: 0.2g
Protein: 6.2g
Carbohydrate: 6.0g

Using a round 5cm diameter crinkle-edged pastry cutter,
cut out rounds of bread from each slice – if you're lucky,
you may get 4 per slice.

Mix together the cream cheese and as many chives as
you wish to use. If it is a little thick, loosen the cheese
with a drop of skimmed milk, but only a drop at a time!

Put the cheese into a small polythene bag and seal the
top. Make a little snip in one corner and you have an
instant piping bag. Pipe rosettes of cream cheese onto
each round – it gets easier with practice! One packet of
cheese should make up to 20 rounds.

Cut the smoked salmon into ribbons and drape a couple over the cream cheese. Separate the onion slices into
individual rings and balance 3 over the salmon. Enjoy!

Tricolour Skewers

Makes about 24

1 pot 200g baby mozzarella balls, each one
   cut in half
1 packet basil leaves
1 punnet baby plum tomatoes or small
   cherry tomatoes, sliced lengthways
50g pesto sauce
light olive oil
salt and freshly ground black pepper
wooden skewers

Info per serving:
Calories: 44.7
Fat: 3.6g
Saturated Fat: 1.3g
Protein: 1.9g
Carbohydrate: 1.4g

Skewer a half-mozzarella ball. Fold a single basil leaf in half and skewer that on top of the cheese. Then spear the tomato lengthways so the three are at the end of the skewer.

In a bowl mix some pesto with some olive oil to loosen it to almost a pouring consistency. When you have completed all the sticks and just before serving, season them. Serve with the bowl of the pesto nearby for dipping.

SKEWERED MEAT, CHICKEN AND FISH

Wooden skewers are great for all sorts of bite-size food for parties.

Using any number of bought marinades, marinate some chicken breasts, beef fillet or fish (tuna, swordfish or monkfish are ideal). Cut into bite-size chunks about 2cm, skewer the meat onto the sticks and grill on a medium heat for a matter of minutes, turning and watching them closely so they don't burn. Pre-soaking the sticks in water for a couple of hours stops them from burning under the grill. Buy a ready-made salsa as a dip for them.

Mange Tout and Prawn Skewers

Makes 20

20 mange tout, boiled for 1 minute then
   plunged into cold water
20 large cooked prawns
small jar of mayonnaise
½ lemon, juiced
wooden skewers

Info per serving:
Calories: 23.4
Fat: 0.3g
Saturated Fat: 0.1g
Protein: 4.8g
Carbohydrate: 0.2g

Pat dry the mange tout so everything is to hand and ready. Hold the prawn in a 'c' shape. Skewer the bottom of the 'c'. Then take a mange tout and, with the skewer, spear a third of the way from underneath to top. Spear the top of the 'c' prawn, then spear just over halfway up the mange tout from the top so the tip of the skewer is hidden behind the vegetable. It will all make perfect sense once you start spearing! Add the lemon juice to the mayonnaise and offer to your non-dieting guests as a dip with their prawns.

FRUIT KEBABS

Use shorter skewers for making fruit kebabs. Steer clear from spearing soft berries such as blackberries or raspberries. Have a chocolate dip at the ready for speared strawberries (again for those nasty non-dieters!). Finish off the skewer with a firm fruit like a grape speared lengthways.

DIPS

All dips should be served with really fresh crudités: peeled and halved celery sticks, peeled carrot sticks, unpeeled seeded cucumber, washed 'breakfast' radishes, baby tomatoes, broccoli and cauliflower florets, and fennel – trimmed and cut into curvy batons.

Red Pepper Houmous

Makes about 300g houmous

1 seeded and roughly chopped red pepper
1 large garlic clove
400g can chickpeas, drained
2 tablespoons light olive oil
1 tablespoon lemon juice
a dash of Tabasco or other 'hot' sauce
salt and freshly ground black pepper

Place the ingredients in a food processor and process until reasonably smooth. Season to taste and chill until needed.

Avocado, Feta Cheese and Tomato

1 large avocado
142ml carton quark
2 spring onions, finely chopped
50g crumbled feta
1 large ripe tomato, seeded and chopped
salt and freshly ground black pepper
Tabasco (optional)

Mash the avocado into the quark. Stir in the onions, feta
and tomato and season with salt and pepper and Tabasco.

Yoghurt, Coriander and Chutney

6 tablespoons mango chutney
small handful of fresh coriander, chopped
4 spring onions, chopped
juice of 2 limes
175g light cream cheese or quark
125g Greek low-fat yoghurt
125g low-fat bio yoghurt
½ teaspoon curry powder
½ teaspoon turmeric
salt and freshly ground black pepper
Tabasco

Blitz everything bar the seasoning in a food processor/blender. Season to taste and chill for at least 30 minutes.

By leaving out the curry powder and adding the same amount of Thai sweet chilli sauce in place of mango chutney, this Indian-style dip becomes a Thai style dip!

Sun-dried Tomato and Cannellini Bean

400g can cannellini beans, drained
8 sun-dried tomatoes in oil, well drained
1 clove garlic, crushed
1 tablespoons light olive oil
2 tablespoons red wine vinegar
125ml water
salt and freshly ground black pepper

Blitz everything except the seasoning in a food processor or blender. If the dip is too thick, add a tablespoon of water at a time for the desired consistency. Season well and chill for at least 30 minutes.

Baby Meringues

Makes 20

These are great 'finger desserts' to round off your buffet or barbeque.

2 egg whites
125g caster sugar
½ teaspoon vanilla extract

Info per serving:
Calories: 27.0
Fat: 0.0g
Saturated Fat: 0.0g
Protein: 2.3g
Carbohydrate: 5.0g

Preheat the oven to 180°C/350°F/Gas mark 4. Line a baking tray with baking parchment. Whip the egg whites in a clean, grease-free bowl until they are stiff and you are brave enough to turn the bowl upside down! Add one spoon of sugar at a time and whisk into the egg white. When all the sugar has been added, the egg whites will be stiff and glossy. Fold the vanilla in with a rubber spatula.

Using two teaspoons put spoonfuls of mixture onto the tray at 2.5cm intervals. Before putting in the oven, make an indent in each meringue using the back of a teaspoon. Bake for 5 minutes and turn down the oven to 120°C/225°F/Gas mark 1 or 2 for 20 minutes. Cool them down completely before removing from the tray.

Fill the meringues with sweetened Greek yoghurt with a little whipped cream added and top with fruit: for example, half a kiwi slice, a raspberry and a few passion fruit seeds or just raspberries and a sprig of mint. Dust with some icing sugar and serve.

BODY BLITZ

JOANNA HALL

Permanent Fat Loss in 5 Simple Steps

Joanna Hall's *Body Blitz* will help you design a diet and fitness program that fits in with your life. This way you can set your own realistic goals – whether you're frazzled with kids, working long hours or simply leading a jam-packed life.

Just follow the 5 steps:

1
Use Joanna's special Starch Curfew® plan
Stop eating certain carbohydrates after 5 pm to boost your energy and lose weight too.

2
Drink a minimum of 2 litres of water a day
This way you'll curb your hunger and enhance your nutrient absorption.

3
Decrease your fat intake
Eat the right fats and see your own body fat decrease.

4
Make time for exercise
Learn how to fit activity into your day.

5
Be consistent – at least 80% of the time
Erratic eating will leave you devoid of energy and prone to putting on the pounds.

Joanna Hall includes a 14-day eating plan, over 25 recipes, and many more ideas for starch-free, low fat meals and snacks. Her program has been tried and tested by real people with real pressures and their own stories and tips will inspire you to win the war against unwanted fat and lack of energy.

CUT THE CARBS AFTER 5PM

JOANNA HALL

Eat the Right Carbs at the Right Time and Lose Fat Fast!

Joanna Hall's Cut the Carbs After 5 pm is both a highly effective and practical diet and fitness plan. It is flexible to fit in with your life, however hectic it is, so that you can maintain your weight loss over the long term.

- How to follow Joanna's Starch Curfew® plan
- Why you should drink 2 litres of water a day
- Why eating the right fats can help your body lose fat
- How to build activity into your day
- Use the 80/20 rule – be consistent 80% of the time

Using these five steps you can really change your level of fitness. And with the delicious selection of Starch Curfew® recipes, you'll lose weight fast.

Make
www.thorsonselement.com
your online sanctuary

Get online information, inspiration and
guidance to help you on the path to physical
and spiritual well-being. Drawing on the integrity
and vision of our authors and titles, and with
health advice, articles, astrology, tarot, a
meditation zone, author interviews and events
listings, www.thorsonselement.com is a great
alternative to help create space and peace
in our lives.

So if you've always wondered about practising
yoga, following an allergy-free diet, using the
tarot or getting a life coach, we can point you
in the right direction.

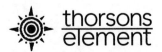

thorsons
element